AF770404

July 1998

Dear Gail,
Words + pictures
heal us.
Keep writing.
In loving kindness,
Rebecca
Sophie

Dear Gail;
A path of compassion
and kindness is
humbling. May our
hearts & souls be
opened by the
courage of those
on a path full
of obstacles.
Warmly,
Katy

An Alphabet about Families Living with HIV/AIDS

Created by
Rebecca Sophia Lee, poet
and
Katy L. Tartakoff, photographer

with
Mary Wilson Blanton
and
Dr. Lori Wiener

Original photographs printed by LeRoy G. Ullmann

Published by
The Children's Legacy
Denver, CO

Funding for
An Alphabet about Families Living with HIV/AIDS
was provided by:

Charleston Area Medical Center, Charleston, WV
DISHES Project, New York City, NY
Gay and Lesbian Fund of Colorado, Colorado Springs, CO
Howard Brown Clinic, Chicago, IL
John M. Lloyd Foundation, Los Angeles, CA
Melvin and Elaine Wolf Foundation, Denver, CO
Anonymous Donor
Anne Avery
Louis Glazer
Stuart Roberts
Shana Stanberry
Suzanne Thorniley
Claire Yaffa

Forward

During the past two decades, HIV infection and AIDS have shattered many of the assumptions and beliefs of health care providers in general and the pediatric care community in particular. For me personally, one of the most remarkable and compelling revelations has been the deepening appreciation of the impact of illness on children and families and, perhaps most notably, the clarity and depth of understanding that children have and express about their experience with illness. They compel us to react to their needs with greater clarity and understanding and, most importantly, with a greater degree of willingness to listen and hear the concerns and messages that they offer to us. Those messages, when received and felt, change our lives and our ability to care successfully for both children and their families.

I applaud the effort of the creators of *An Alphabet about Families Living with HIV/AIDS* in bringing the lives of children and families with HIV infection to us. The book personalizes the impact of this disease and reaches out to touch our hearts and souls, as well as our minds and intellects. Pictures of families coupled with the voices of their words remind us of who we are and what our mission is about. We are here to serve and to care for families and, for some of us, through our science, to improve their lives through new treatments and preventative strategies.

Regardless of our calling and the skills we bring to bear, *An Alphabet about Families Living with HIV/AIDS* also serves as a mirror reflecting the subtle lines that connect us as either patients or providers. One day all of us will cross that line and look back at our providers with the hope that they will be as aware of our feelings as they are of our bodies. *An Alphabet about Families Living with HIV/AIDS* reminds us of that connectedness and calls each of us to join hands now as we look and listen to the living portrait that our children and families present to us.

Philip A. Pizzo, M.D.
Harvard Medical School
Department of Pediatrics

Children's Hospital of Boston
Department of Medicine

An Alphabet about Families Living with HIV/AIDS
was made possible by the assistance and support
of the following people and organizations:

Boston, MA
Dr. Sandra Bertman
Kathie Hartnett
Nancy King-Bolger
Michelle Papazian
Dr. Phil Pizzo
Jasmine Quazilbash
Peter & Amy Tartakoff
Julie Wechstein
Boston Children's Hospital
Midwest Express Airlines

Denver/Boulder, CO
Rita Berglund
Brad Droy
Joanne Elliot
Patti Held
Lorie Hirose
Gary & Elizabeth Jones
Mary Ladd
Kathy Nuanes
Patti Pedden
Laura Pritchard-Haile
Amanda Rosas
Ron Schimmel
Michael Simon
Phoebe Sophocles
Dr. Charles Steinberg
LeRoy Ullmann
Marianne Weiner
Nina Williams
Janice Woods
Toba Zaritsky
AIDS, Medicine and Miracles
Angels Unaware
Children participating in Legacy
Workshops Summer 1996
The Children's Hospital HIV Clinic
Denver Art Museum
Denver General Hospital ID Clinic
Denver Museum of Natural History
Droy Advertising
Eron Johnson Antiques, Ltd.
Kodak
M Gallery
Resolute
The Travel Society

Grand Rapids, MI
A. James Heynen
Jill Novak
Family AIDS Network
The Greystone Group

Las Vegas, NV
Pat Broadbent
Reach Out

Los Angeles, CA
Scott Barton
Bill Bingham
Aileen Getty
Steven Grissom
Herb Hamsher
D.H. Lewis
Judith Light
Sharon Lund
Sarah Michel
Suzie Zeegen

New York, NY
Anne Cullen
Milton Esterow
Scott Hirose

San Diego, CA
Dr. Jerome Sattler

San Francisco, CA
Lucy Barnett
Susan & Harry Dennis
Barbara Shoolery
VNA & Hospice of Northern
California

Seattle, WA
Jeri Easler
Wendy Forselius
Val Piacenti
Janet Trinkhaus
Jenny Vonckx
Rise N' Shine

Washington, D.C.
Children participating in clinical
trials in the HIV & AIDS
malignancy branch of the
National Cancer Institute
Children enrolled in the National
Cancer Institute's Pediatric
HIV/AIDS Clinic
Ellen Townley
Dr. Lauren Wood
CDC Clearing House

Chiang Mai, Thailand
Jane Arnott
Rev. Lauren Bethell
Kim Brown
Kathleen Dugan
Dr. Vicharn Vithayasai
Faye Wimonsuksuwan
Agape House
Chiang Mai Hospital
House of Love
The New Life Center

We dedicate this book

to the children and families we have been honored to know,
with appreciation for your teachings, wisdom and inspiration.

to our own families who have made this journey with us.

to our many friends who are living through the tragedy of AIDS
and have provided enormous insights along the way.

to all those whose faces and names remain invisible
but whose voices are hopefully heard in the poems
and felt within the photographs.

to those who are no longer here.

Introduction

We, the creators of *An Alphabet about Families Living with HIV/AIDS,* are mothers, daughters, photographers, writers and artists who treasure the healing power of stepping forward and naming our truth. One of us is HIV positive and has lost a spouse to AIDS and a baby because of AIDS. Another, a social worker, has been on the front line of the HIV epidemic since the early days in New York when gay men began appearing in emergency rooms with a life-threatening form of pneumonia. Our photographer has been making images of families living with HIV/AIDS for ten years, and our poet has been writing poetry and nonfiction for nine years, the majority of it rooted in life with a handicapped daughter. We have been moved to tell the stories, through words and images, of a group of families living with HIV. By giving them voice, we hope to give voice to the thousands of families across the globe living with AIDS.

We were committed to publishing images that applaud the human spirit and celebrate the miracle of life. We did not wish to show people dying from AIDS, but rather wanted to portray families living with a virus that poses a daily threat to life as they know it. We wanted to honor their struggle with isolation, stigma, and discrimination and, at the same time, capture the joy of loving and being loved by family.

Our message to the reader living with HIV, or loving and caring for someone living with HIV, is heartfelt. Our wish is that you see something in a photograph, or feel something when you read a poem, that mirrors your struggle and your dreams, and tells a piece of your story. We welcome you to join these pages in spirit. And if you know others who might feel a healing connection with the faces and the words, please share the book with them.

We ask the readers not living with HIV to consider the multiple losses in families where one or more members is living with and most probably will one day die from AIDS. The number of children worldwide who know the depth, sorrow and impact of the loss of loved ones is nothing short of staggering, and the numbers are growing.

As we met and photographed families for the book, we were moved so many times by the creative and loving ways in which new families are formed, or those in existence are made larger, to care for children who have lost parents, siblings, aunts and uncles. This willingness to take in others who were not born to us, or to raise a second generation when our own children have died, is life-affirming and precious. It is a selfless act of doing what needs to be done. It is an act of love. And for all its devastation and heartbreak, this disease is surrounded by acts of love.

This book is a format for families to leave a legacy for loved ones. Each photograph contains at least one person living with HIV/AIDS. There are people in the book who have died in the interim between photography and publication. Other families have not been public with their disease until now. The families were asked to comprise a list of words for each letter of the alphabet. From adults and children who live with the emotional and physical wounds of a disease both terminal and isolating, came Hope, the word submitted more frequently than all others.

With the advent of protease inhibitors, many people infected with HIV are living longer and living better, but the drugs are expensive and not everyone benefits from the treatment, nor can everyone tolerate the side effects. Disappointingly, a drug will work for a period of time and then lose its effect in a particular individual. A cure continues to elude us and, as of publication, there is no vaccine to protect the uninfected. Until a cure is found, we encourage you to do what you can to end the pandemic scope of AIDS, and to heal its wounds of isolation and loneliness.

April 1998

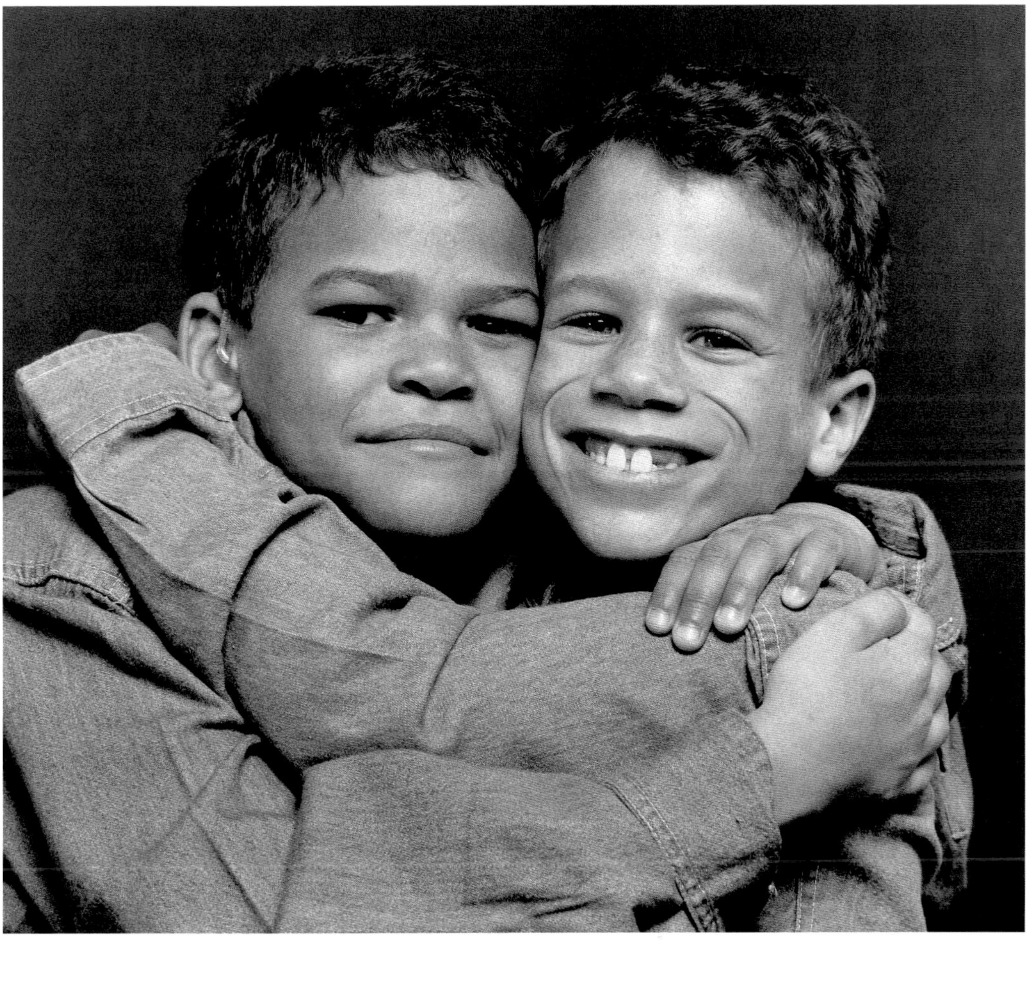

A

AIDS . . .
at home among us,
a contorted ally,
an alien who lands
anywhere, with anyone,
anytime.

I ask you,
would the Almighty
feel as alone
as I, as angry,
afraid and abandoned
as I who want
to slay this monster
named AIDS?

what if
a pair of wings
sprouted through the cotton of
your favorite t-shirt and
flew you into the arms
of a guardian angel.
what if?

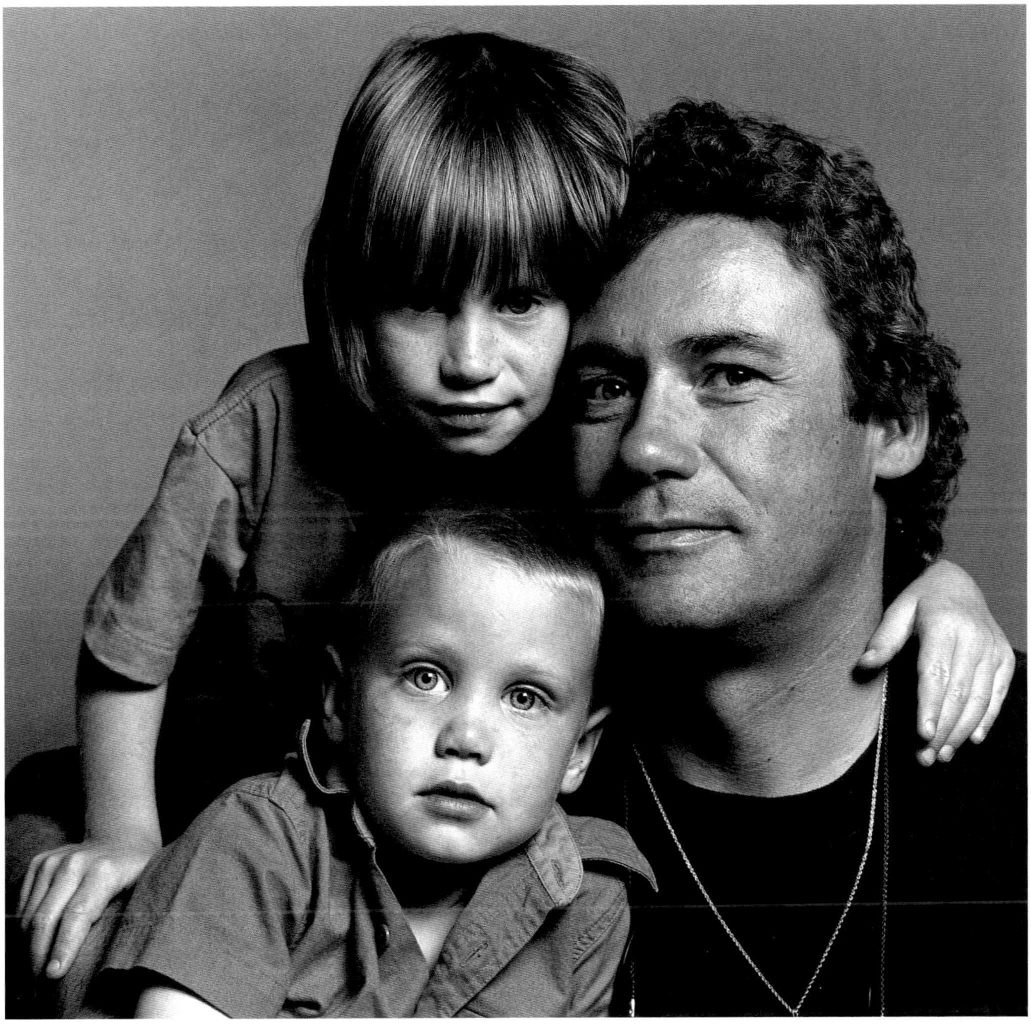

A

I crawl out
from the deepest part,
my alcove of agony,
awestruck and grateful
that I have not forgotten
how to appreciate
all that I am.

reaching into my bones,
into the marrow of me,
I ask why
and then remember that
why will never be answered,
that the most I can ask for
is acceptance.

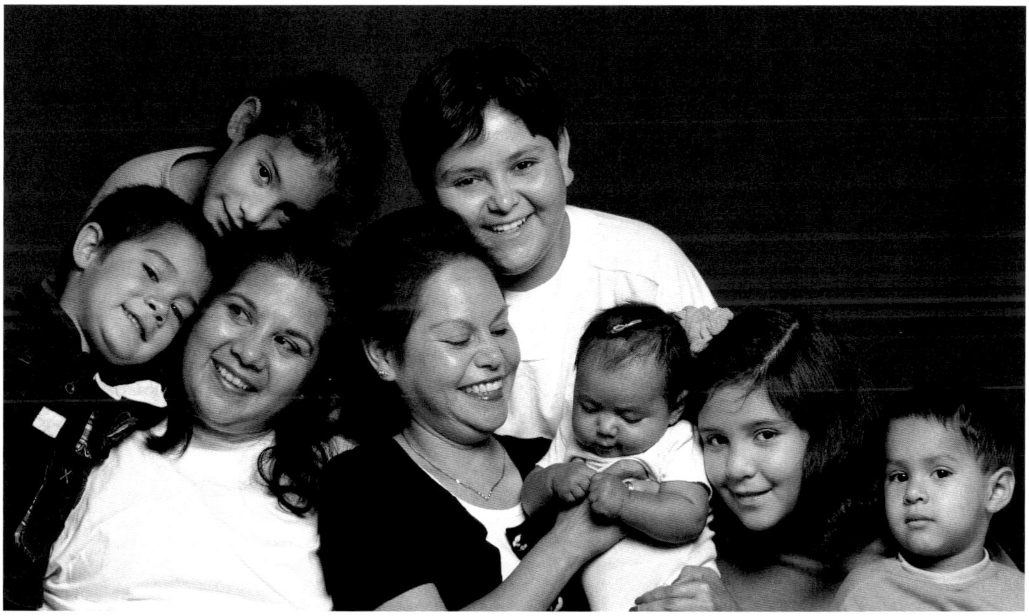

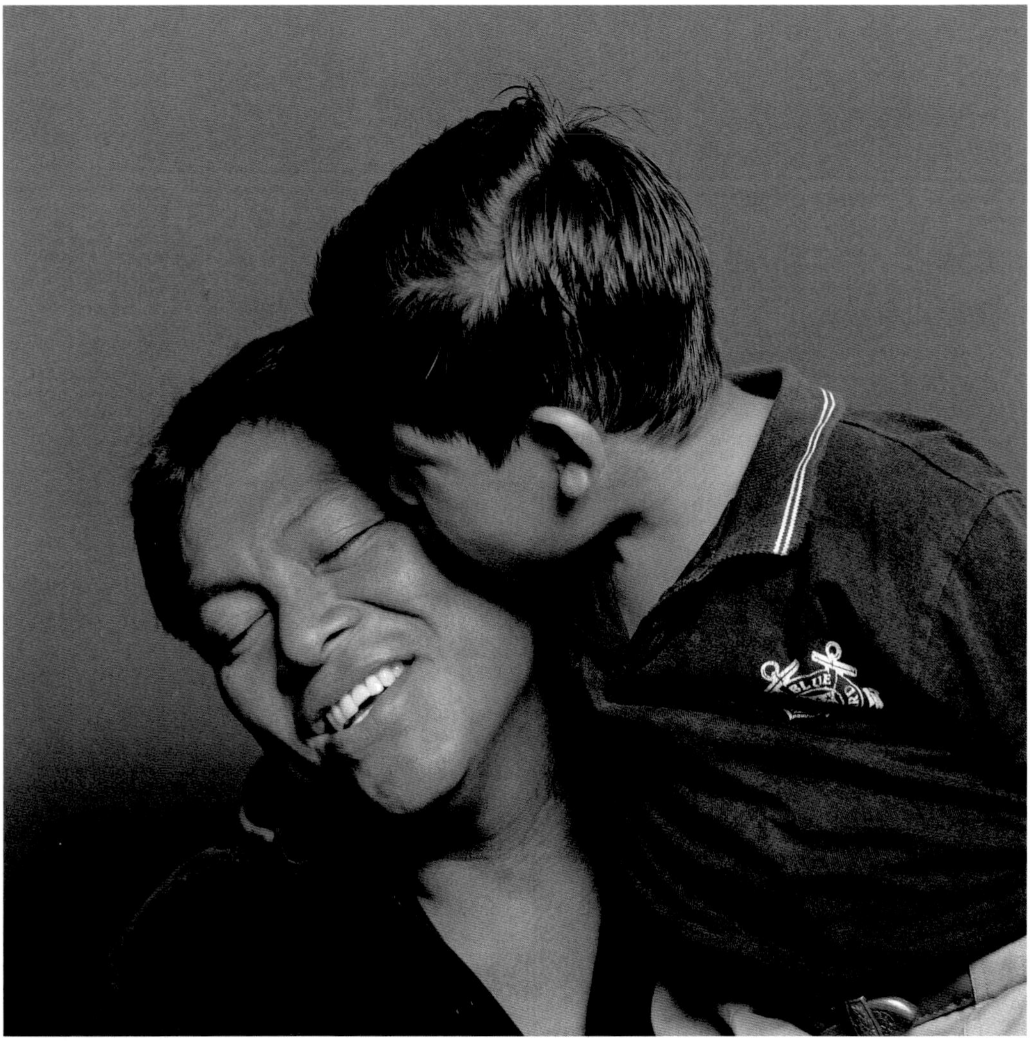
BLUE

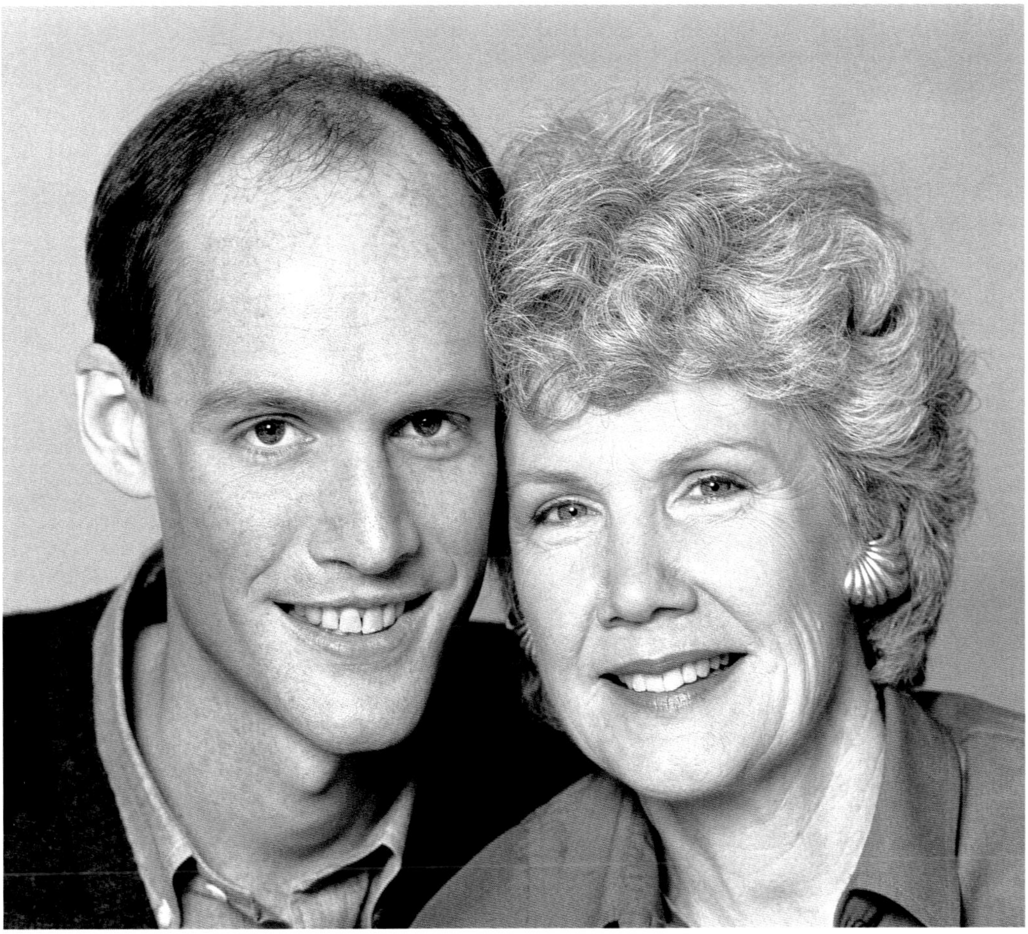

B

betrayed before she took
her first breath,
my baby is a bird
named grace who lands
on my shoulder and in her sweet
whisper, reminds me
to count my blessings
to live my truth.

do not advise me to be
thankful for every minute
as I sit in dis-belief
over broken blood, the bearer
of this bothersome dis-ease
that makes it hard to be brave.

HIV is a burden
we bear with the spirit
of a black stallion,
bold and beautiful,
all the while
baffled by the notion
of invisible blessing.

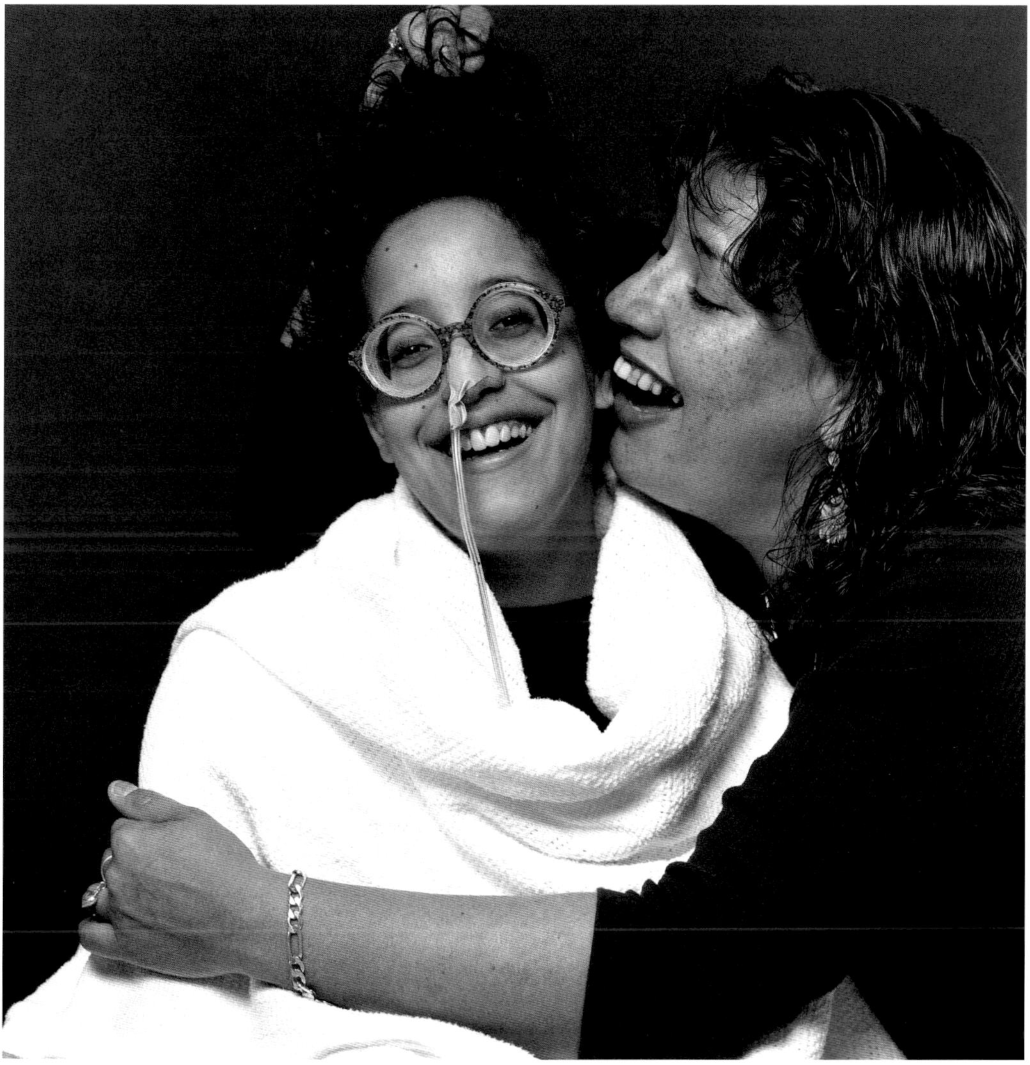

C

color your courage
a rainbow, curious
child, and celebrate
each dawn
that comes into
a culture unable
to find a cure.

the clinic is a crazy
community of comrades
and caregivers, a common
place where confusion
sits next to courtesy,
where air grows sour
with the stench of anxiety,
the clatter of a cough
blends with the chill
of cancer, and a cut
is cause for chaos.

hear the cry of compassion
as the caregiver turns her back
and wipes a tired face
against her sleeve of pastel cotton.

comfort comes
when you tell me
we are in this together.

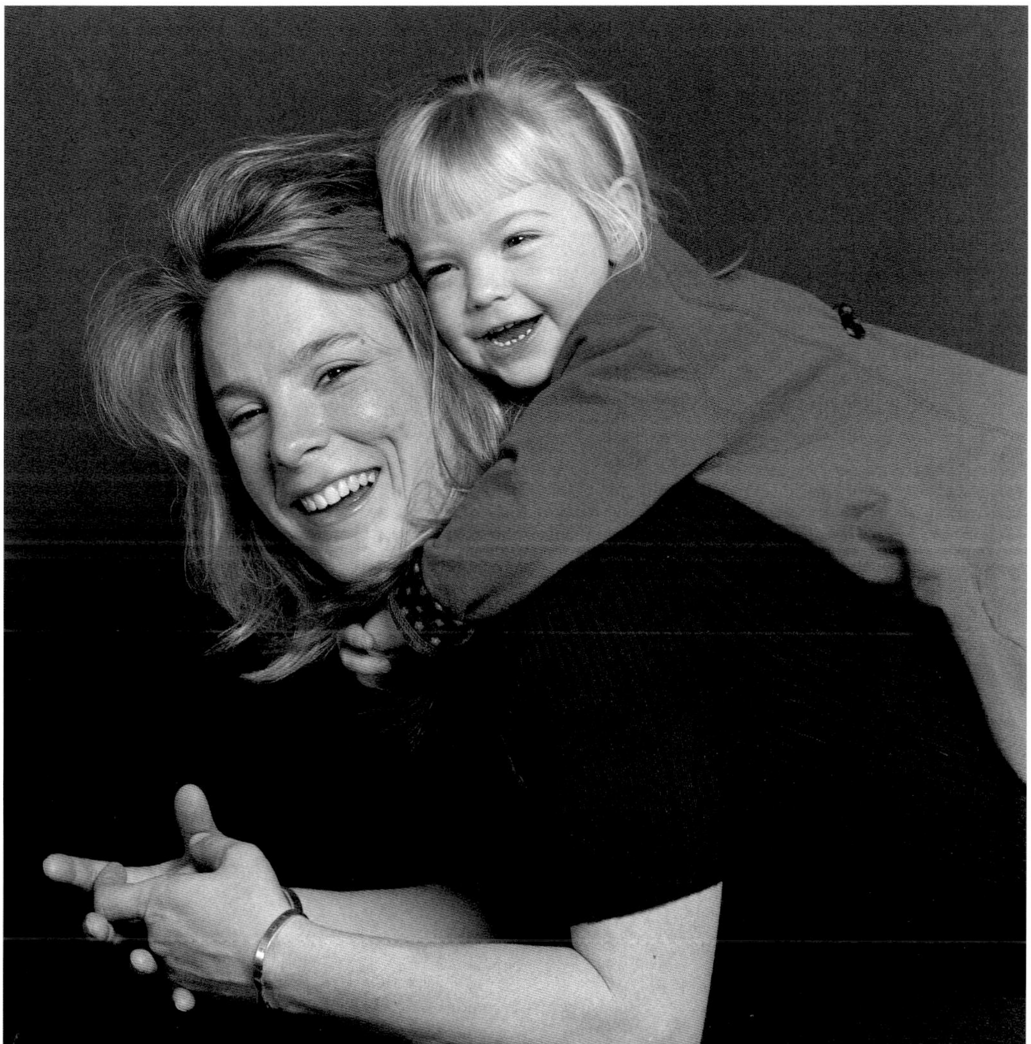

D

a disease named AIDS
has neutralized our diversity
and compressed our differences
into the single moment
common to us all:
the moment of disclosure.

of all the demands
this disease has dropped
at my feet, the hardest
is preparing a place where
your questions will be heard,
your anger understood,
your dreams nurtured and
my memory preserved.

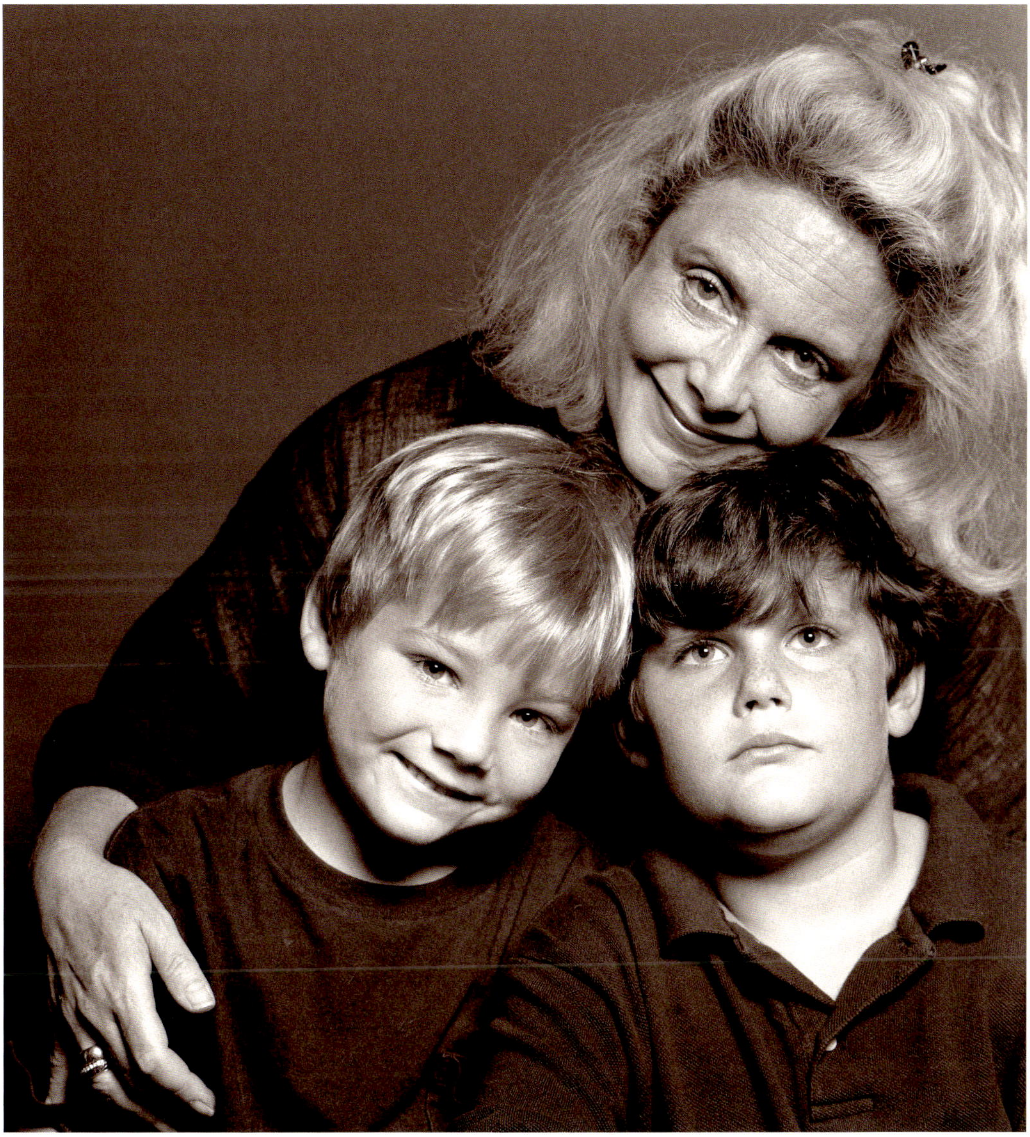

D

we stand tall
at death's door,
determined that our
departure be different
from friends who denied
the devastation of this despicable
disease and flirted
with disaster.

we march in solidarity
defying the pronouncement
we wear as a halo
our scarlet A
and delight in day-to-day
life with dignity.

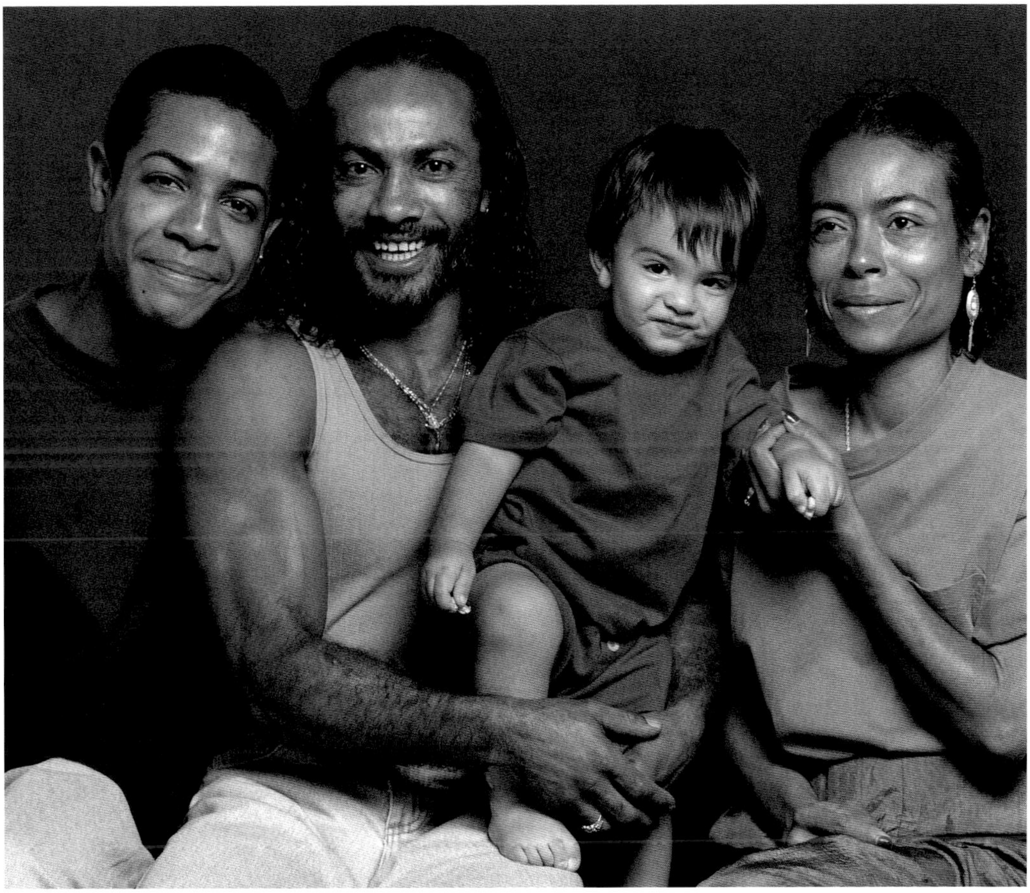

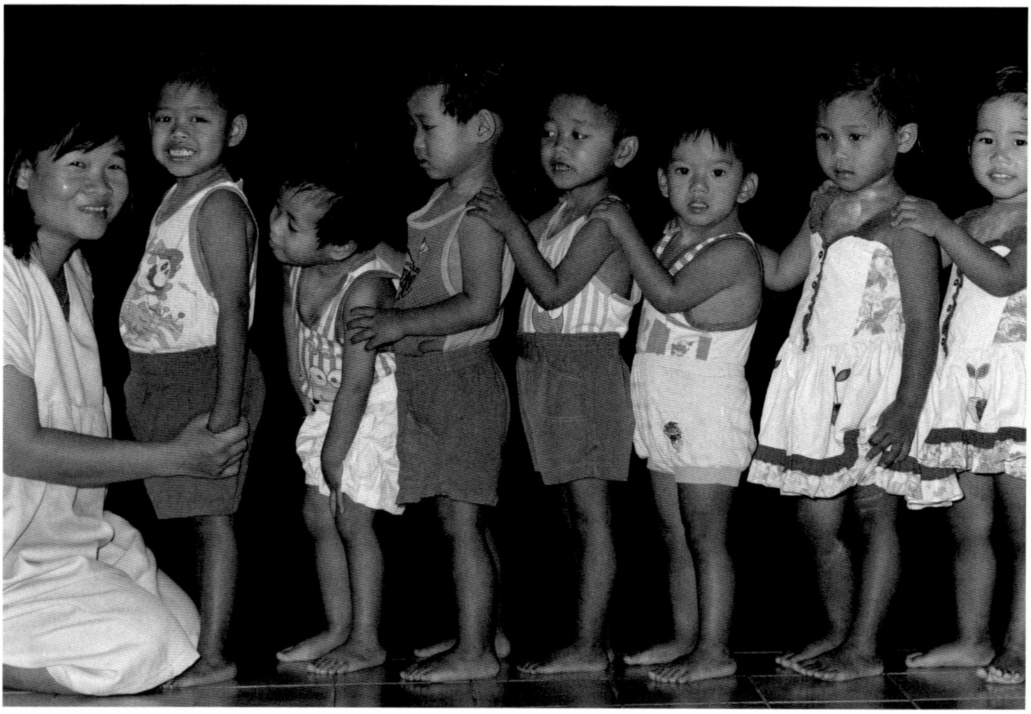

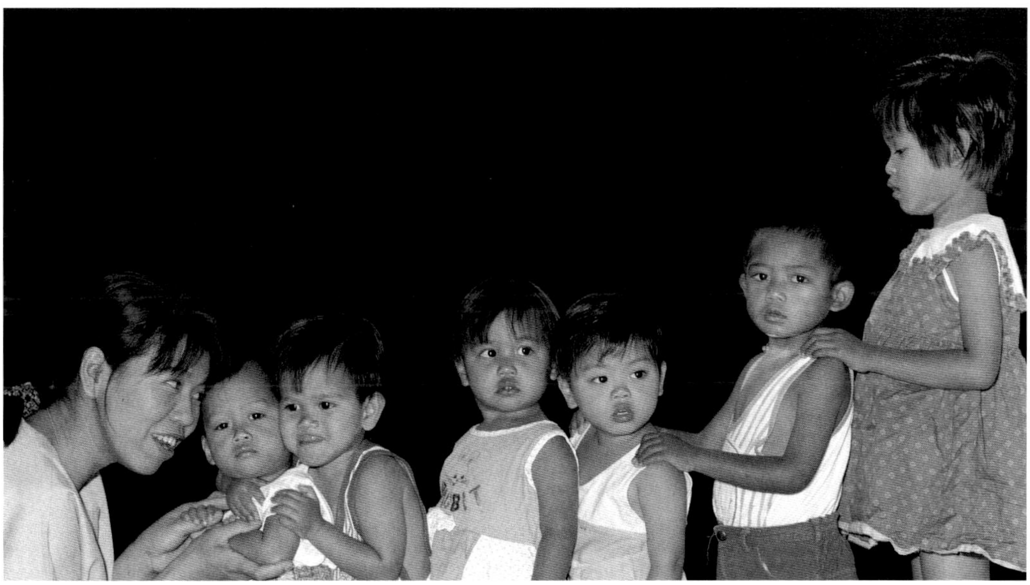

E

take one deep
breath and remember that
nothing happens
without effort.

this global enemy
undefeated is
everyone's emergency,
everyone's error,
everyone's evil.

AIDS . . . you elephant!
teaching us daily
to endure the embarrassment,
to enjoy what is.

eliminate this epidemic
of exhaustion and envy,
end our need for
an early eulogy.

wrap my fingers
around the AIDS escape hatch
and hear me exhale
in eloquent relief!

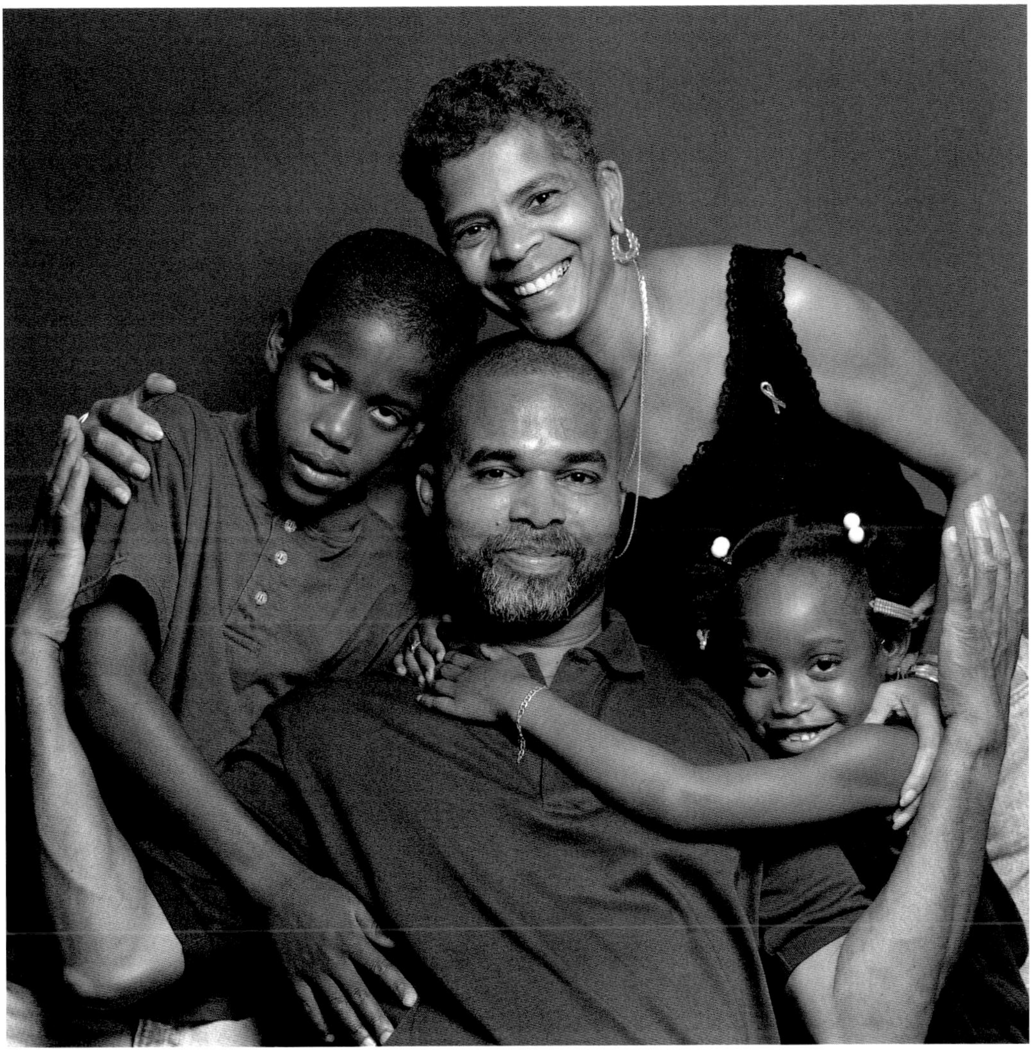

F

a fatal fungus
steals my future
as if she were a lit
match dropped upon
a bed of straw,
the fairy tale without
a princess and I,
in failed flight,
frightened by the fallacy
that anything, anybody,
could possibly last
forever.

one of the gifts
are the adopted families
created to care
for the angels who stay.

freedom
is a phantom
I once knew
as friend.

faith has become
a family heirloom
wrapped in silk,
hidden in a fancy
box filled with
faces of forgiveness.

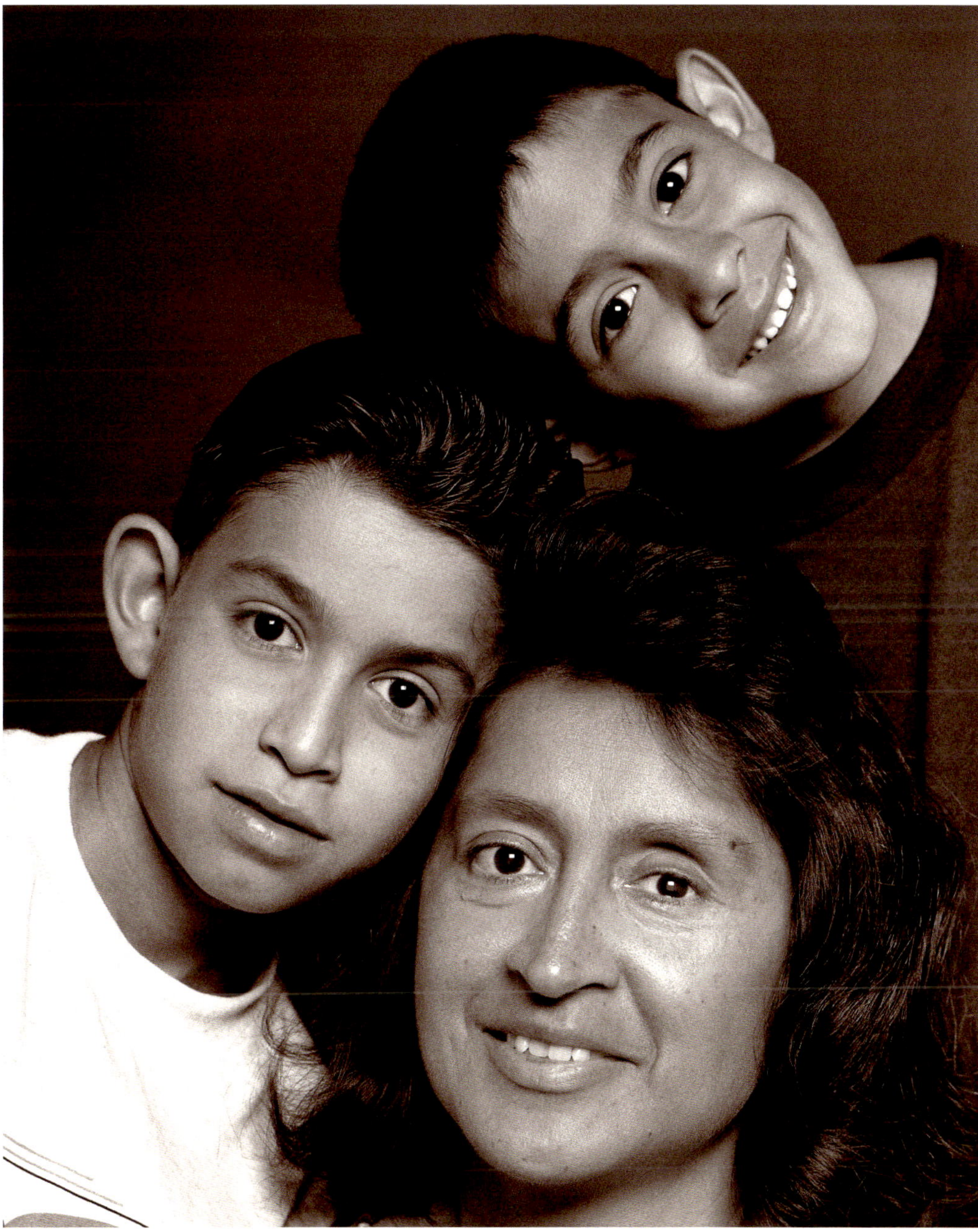

G

a gentle God
is loving me through
this lifetime of good
days numbered.

grief lays over me
like grandmother's quilt,
meticulously sewn from
squares of mismatched
fabric whose worn
threads weave
a patchwork of grace.

the gusto required
to pour weeks of life
into every day
has me grumpy, has me scared
that one day the grace and
the guilt will be gone.

good friends
on bad days
are gifts
from God.

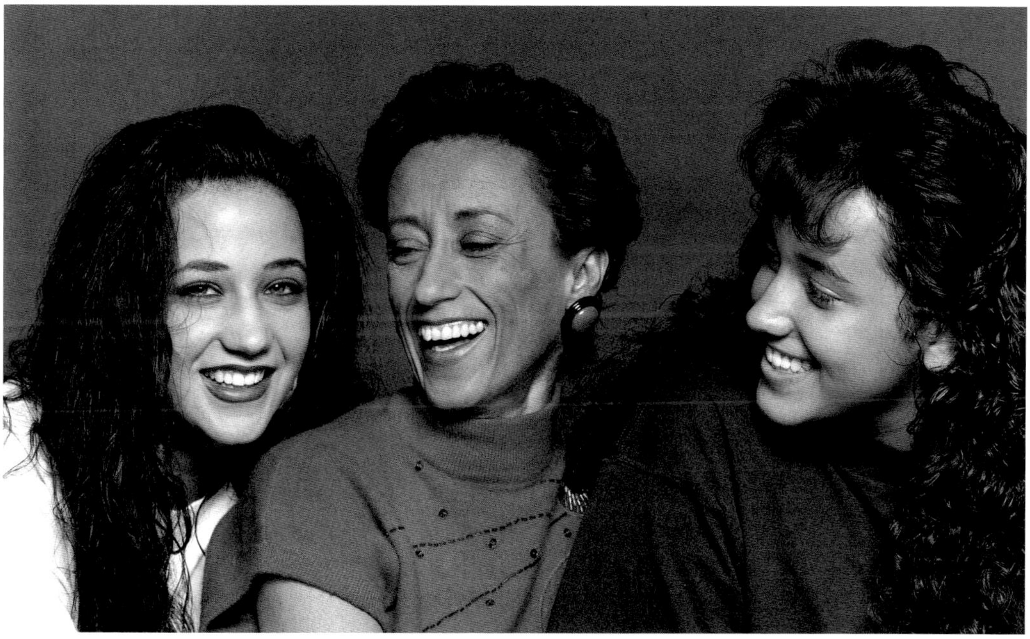

H

holding
kissing
hugging
touching . . .
still safe,
forever heavenly.

we hate hiding
the truth . . . honestly.
our hearts are blue
from holding our breath
in hopes of healing
before you learn
who we are.

as if HIV
were not enough,
now I must tell you that
I have herpes and
enter once again
the horrific hell that
blows my cover
each time I pretend
to have found a safe place.

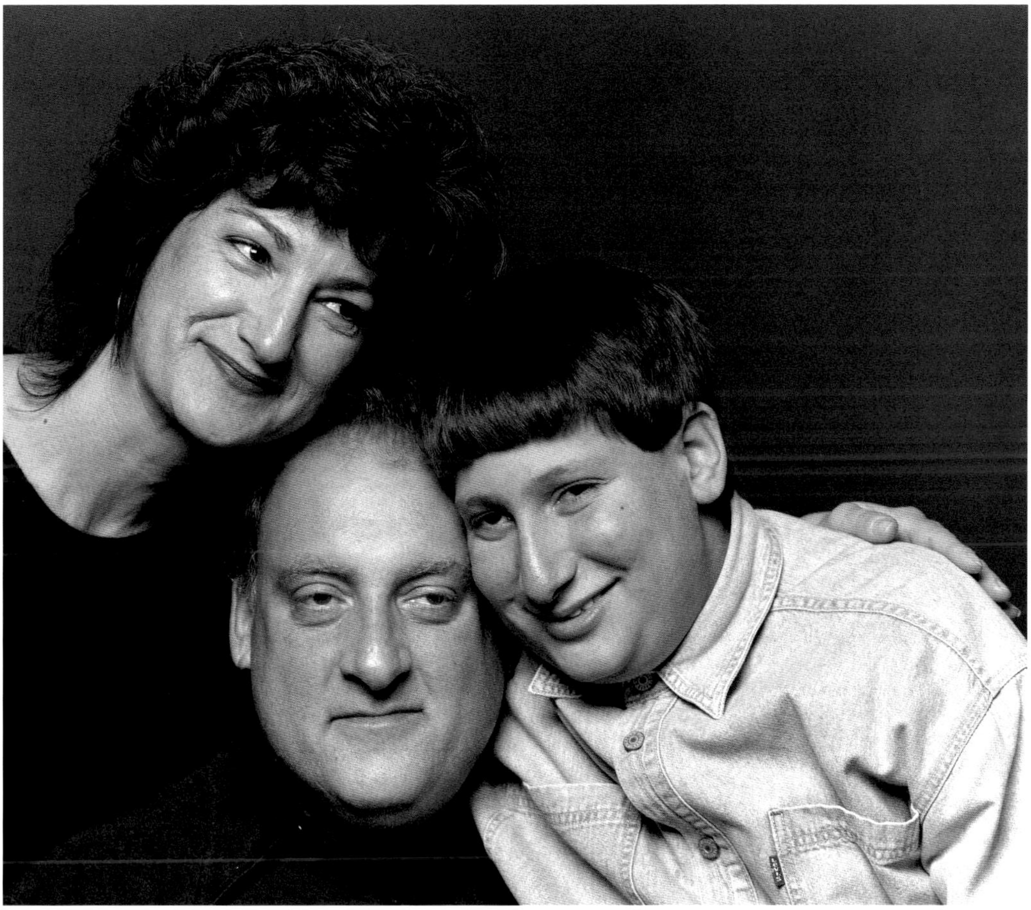

I

isolation
prohibits me
from giving you
inspiration.

this intimate disease reminds us
of the instability of life
and injects our calloused hearts
with gentleness as we exchange ignorance,
judgment, fear and resentment
for a generous dose of compassion.

if my illness
were invisible,
would you insult
me less?

ignorance
offers less immunity
than an inquisitive
intelligence.

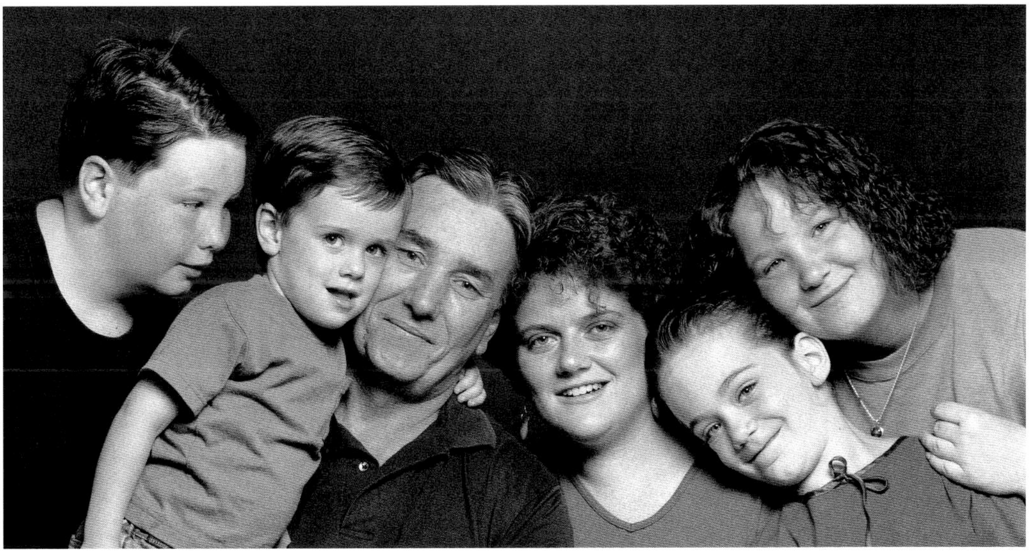

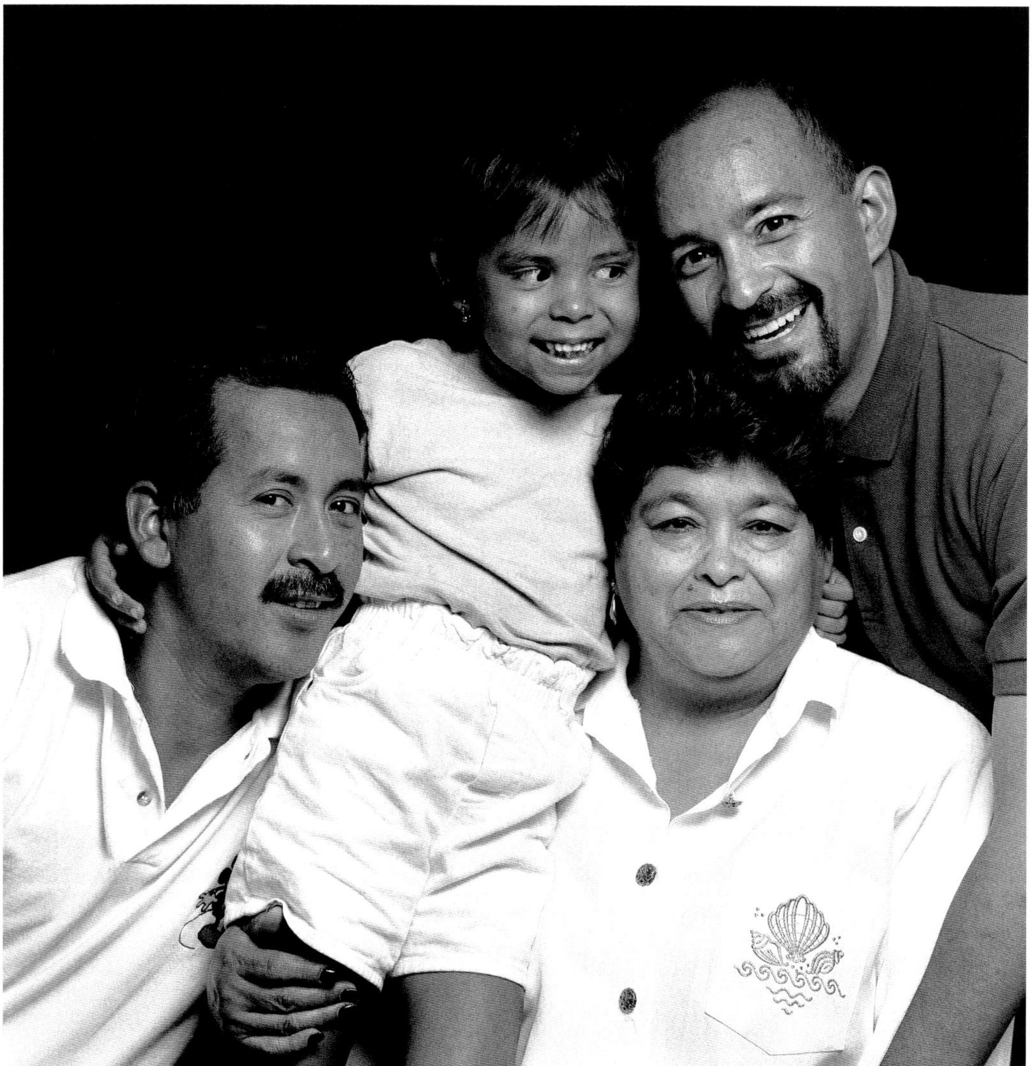

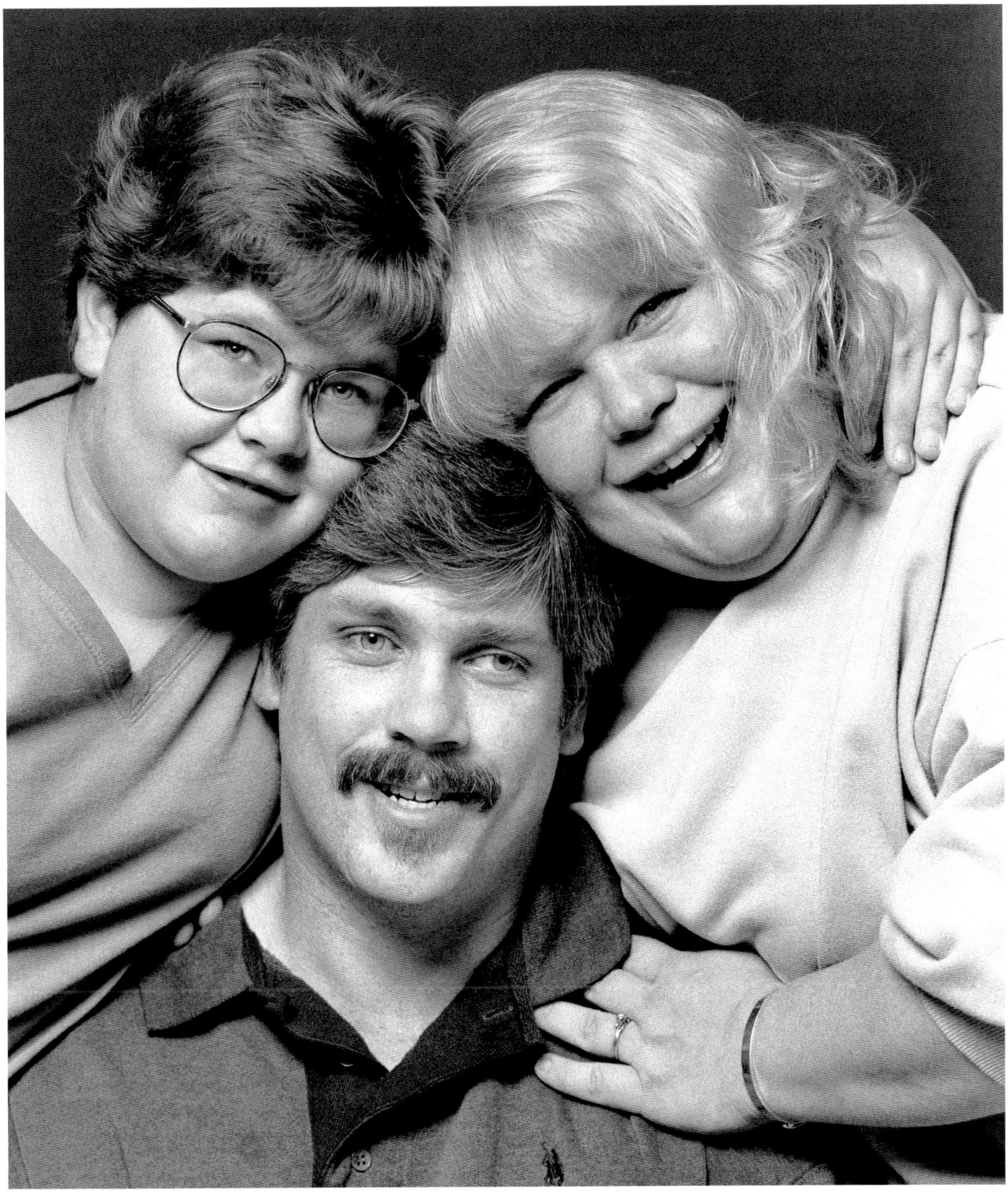

J

a jackal
unseen
untouched
and
invincible
has placed
my life
in jeopardy.

beware
the judgments
made on
our journey
to stay
alive,
warns the jokester.

just once
I wish
these pills
tasted
sweet as
jellybeans.

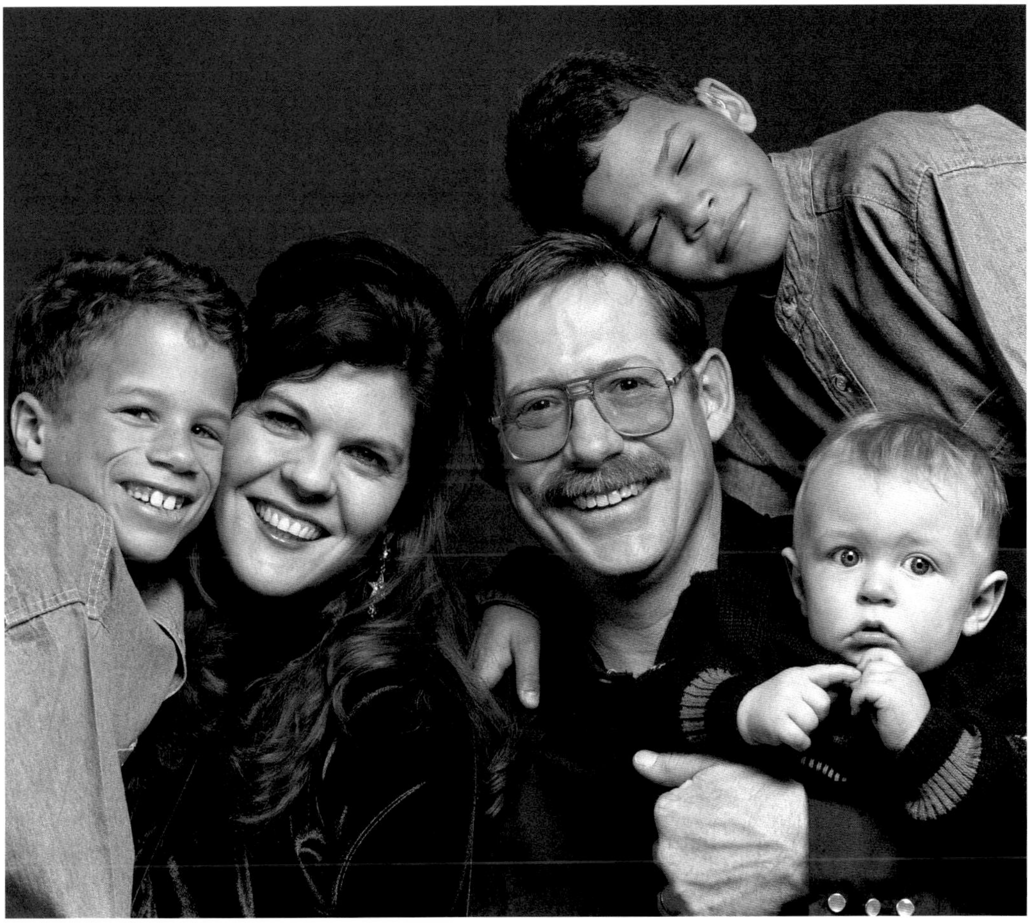

K

if you knew my secret
about this killer virus
would you hoard your kindness
in your kangaroo pouch,
or would you kiss my cheek,
hold my cold
hand and keep me
forever in your heart?

kaput
karma
keep
key
kids
kill
killer
kindless
kind
kisses
knowing

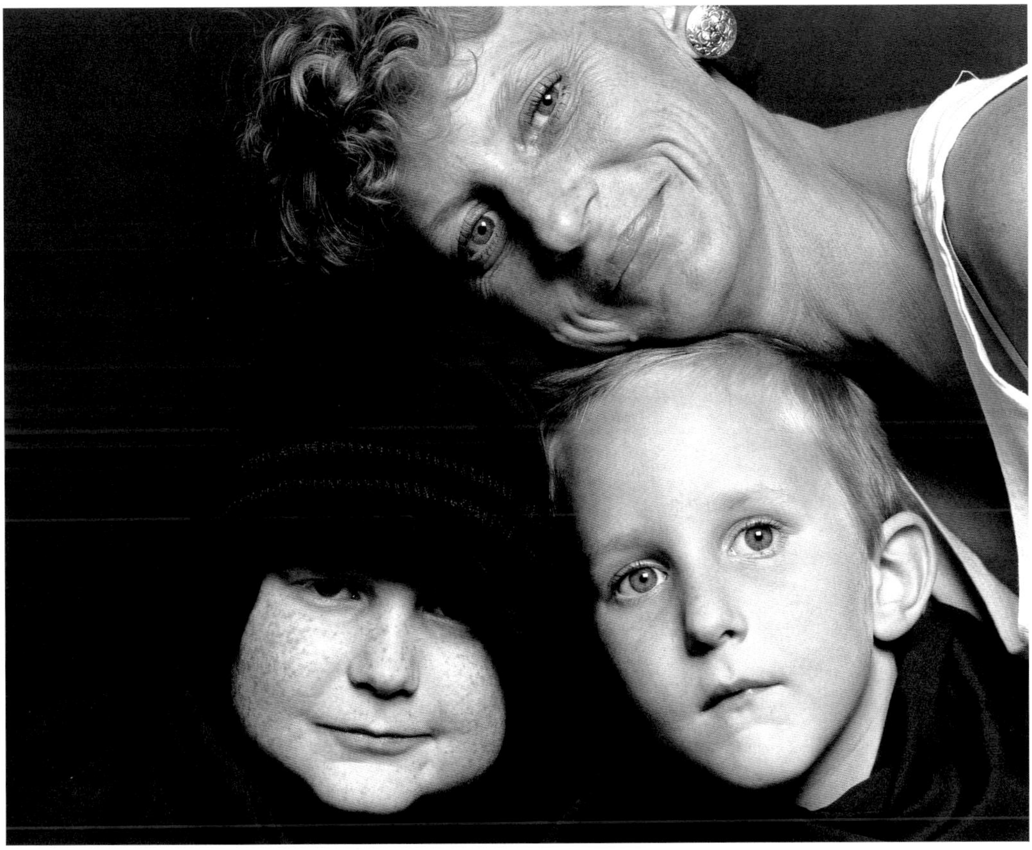

L

loving my family
transforms the loneliness
of living with AIDS
into a lioness whose roar
quiets the boasting
of those who believe
this limited lifetime
could never happen
to them.

we
who are
on this side of
lonesome
love
without
limit.

when I go
I have not
left.
hear me
laughing
and remember
my love.

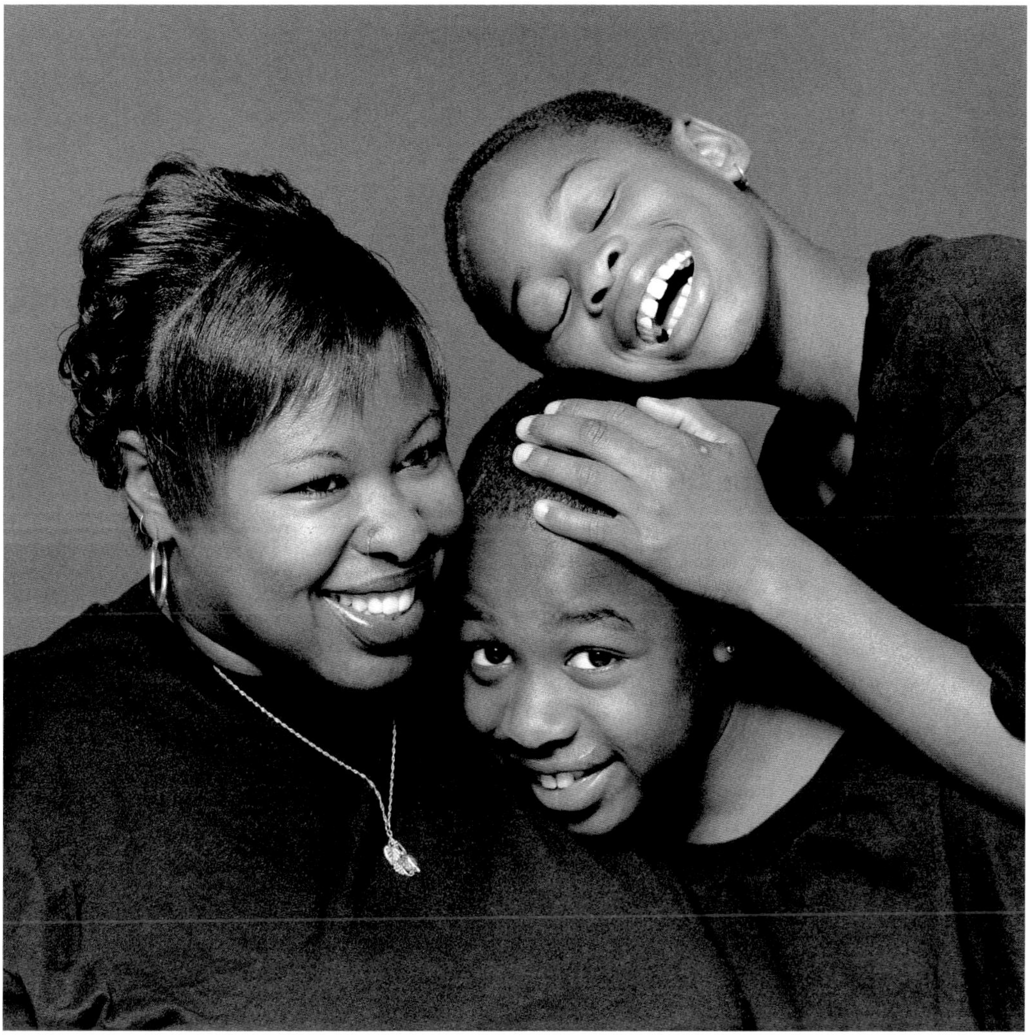

M

days, weeks,
precious months are infused
with this manic urge
to feel every tickle
life has to give,
to miss nothing as
the monkey called AIDS
marches up my spine and
sinks into my bones.

one could go mad
making friends
with the experimental mass
spread across
my kitchen table.

when you look in the mirror,
hold no malice . . .
it will only make you miserable.

life is made up of
moments
methodology
misery
mystery
malice
mourning
magic
and
miracles.

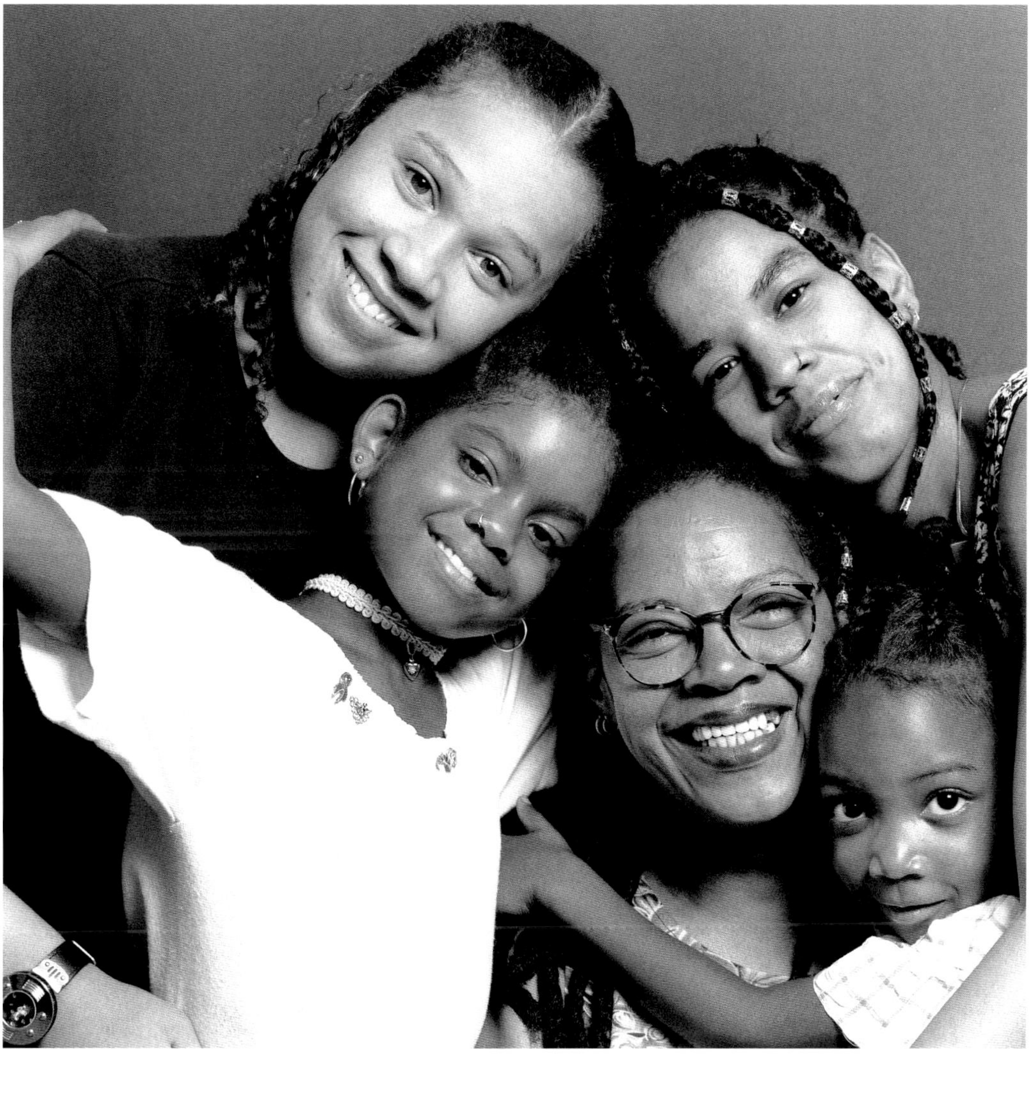

N

new findings
new treatments
new medicine
new pills
new hope
same disease
old nightmare.

practice feeling
nourished by needles
or cleansed by nausea and
you will understand
my never ending
scream . . . NO!
NOT YET!

now that the nurses
have made me promise
to never say never,
I need to take
a nap.

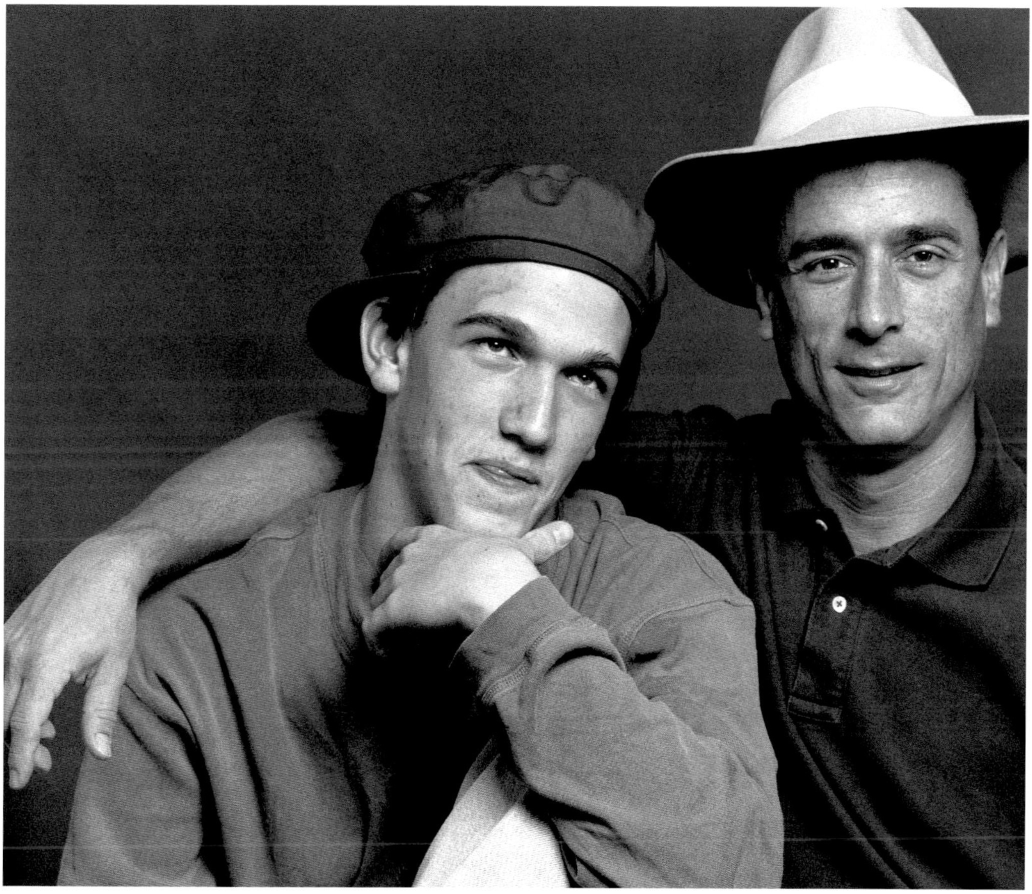

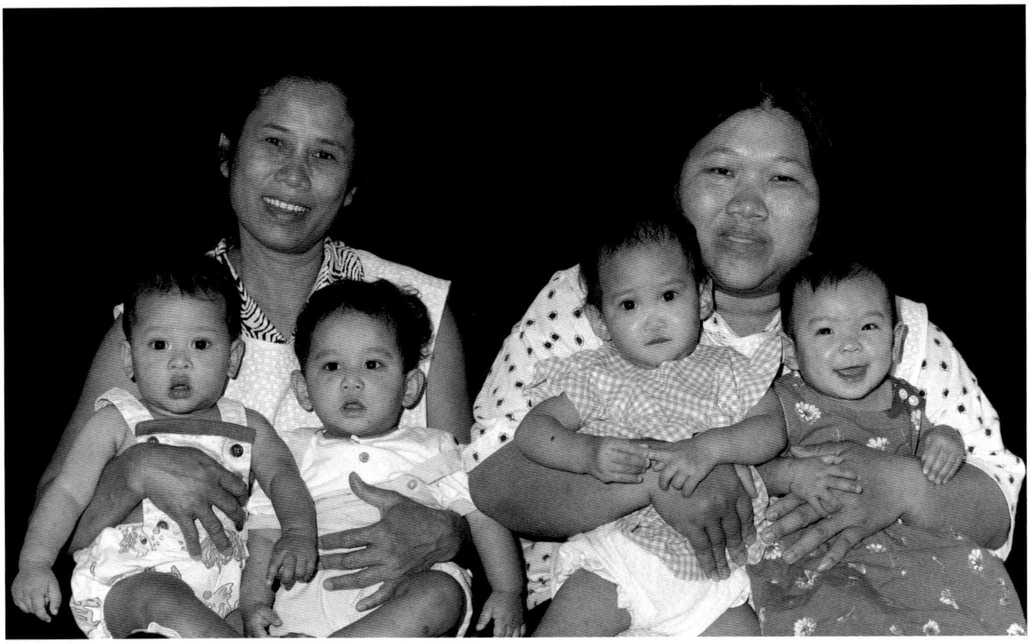

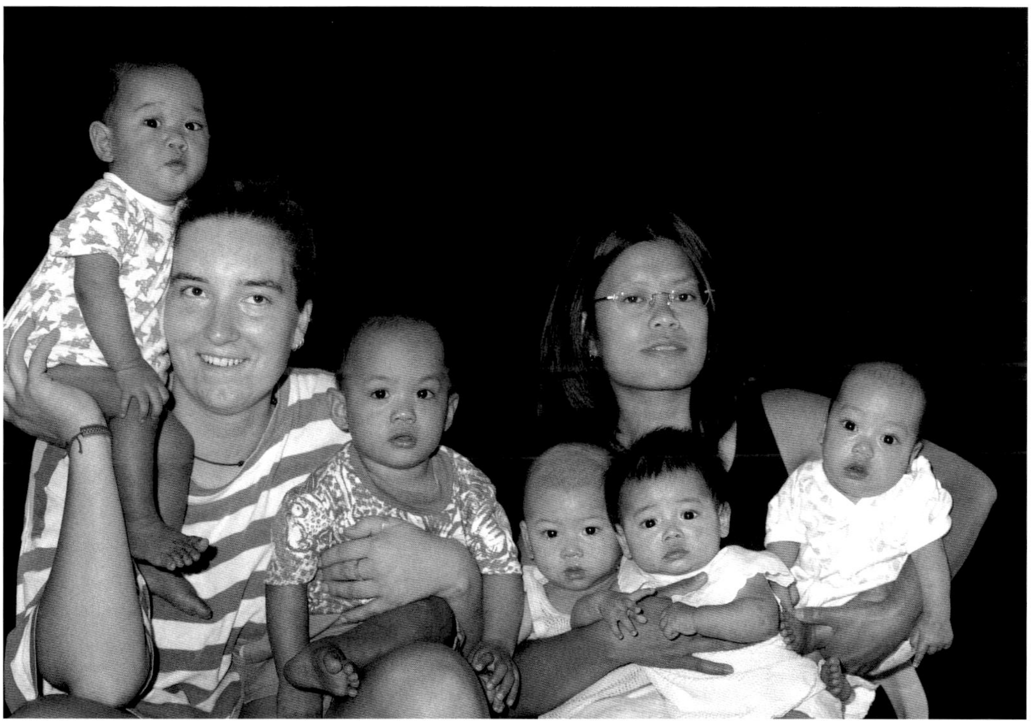

O

own opinions
that open your heart
instead of opinions that
isolate
and
oppress.

I am an outpatient
in search of
an oasis where
no one hollers
OUCH!

when the time
comes
think of me
in a room
on the other
side of a
locked
door that will
one day
open.

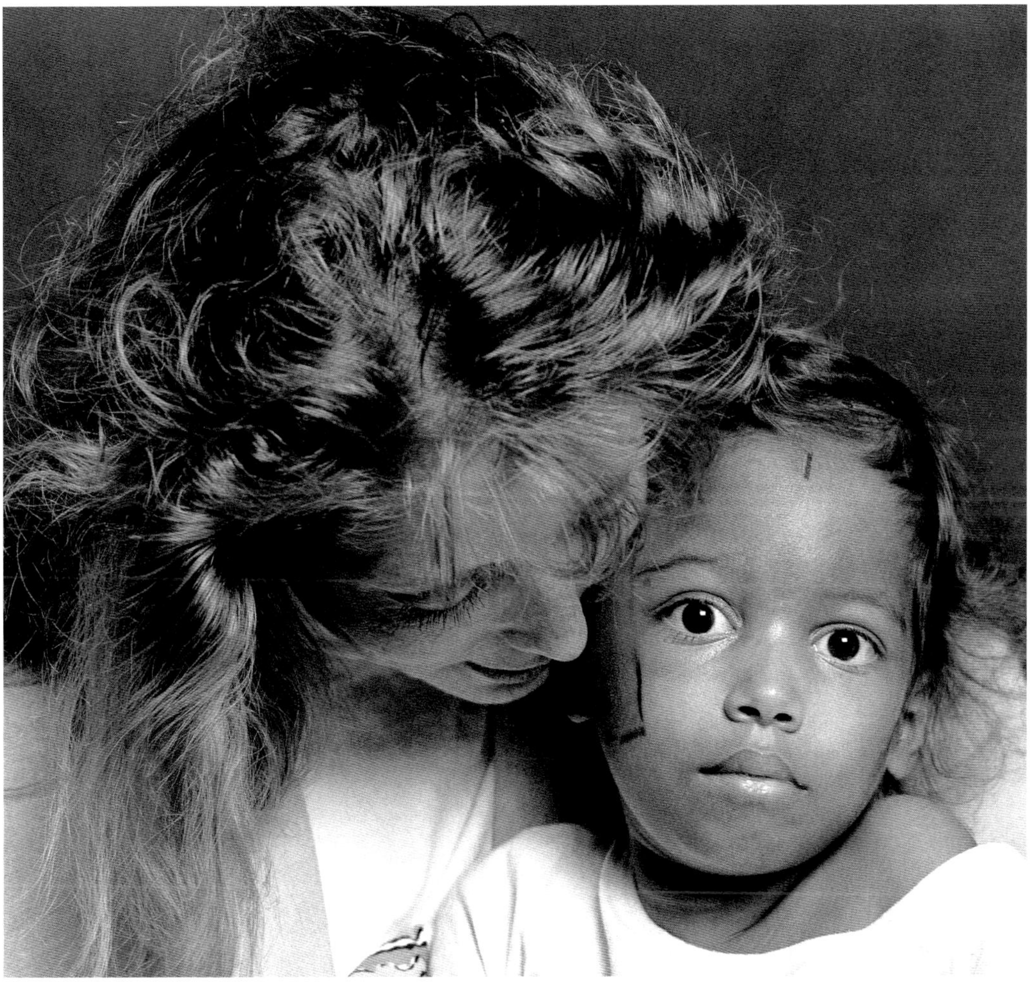

P

I pray
for the peace
that AIDS
interrupted.

dear physician,
can you promise this
poke will not hurt?
dear pharmacist,
does your bag of pills
contain any protection
from my prognosis?

is protease inhibitor
a pro
come to save us
or a bully
come to tease?

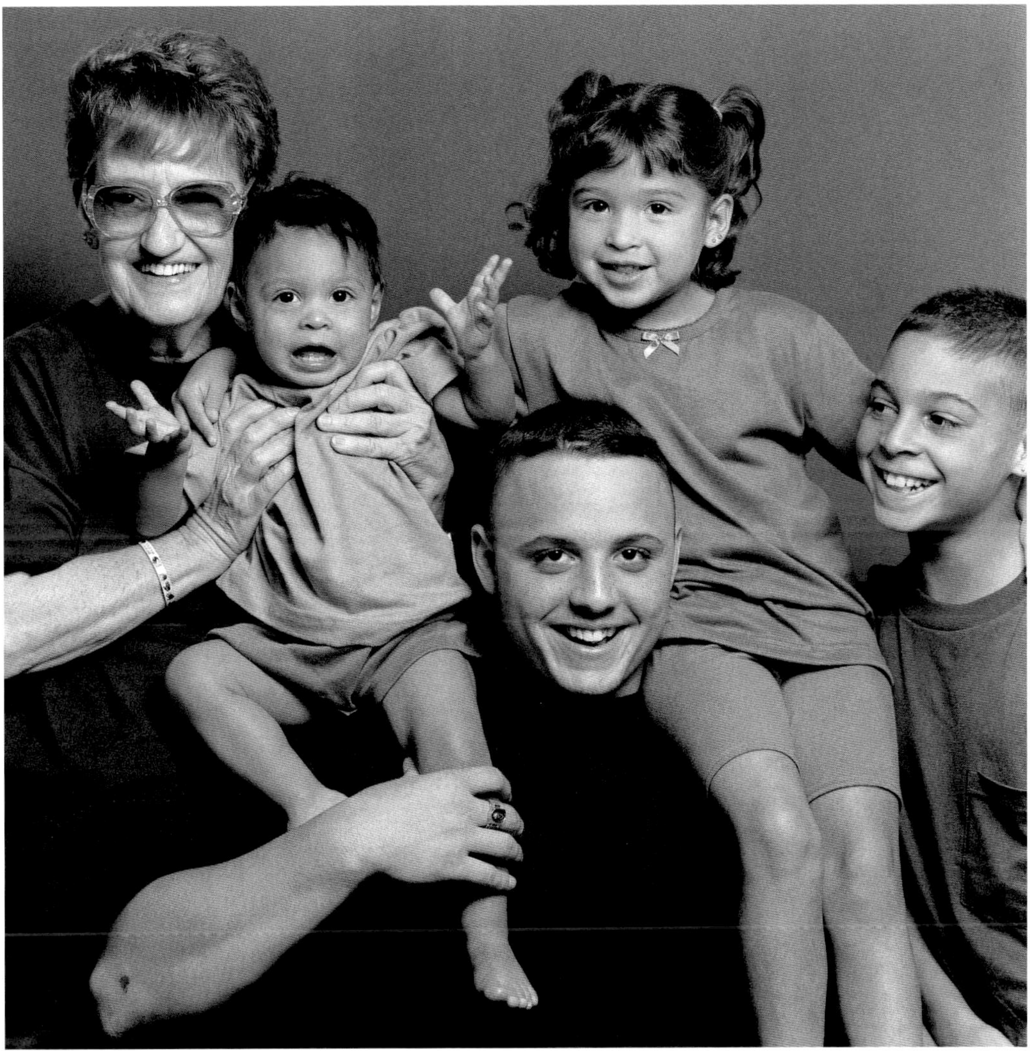

P

a promise –
I will not leave you,
I will always love you,
help you, and never
forget you –
a promise.

we are prisoners
without stripes
serving time
on a precarious
pilgrimage of
protocol
patience
perspective
power
peace.

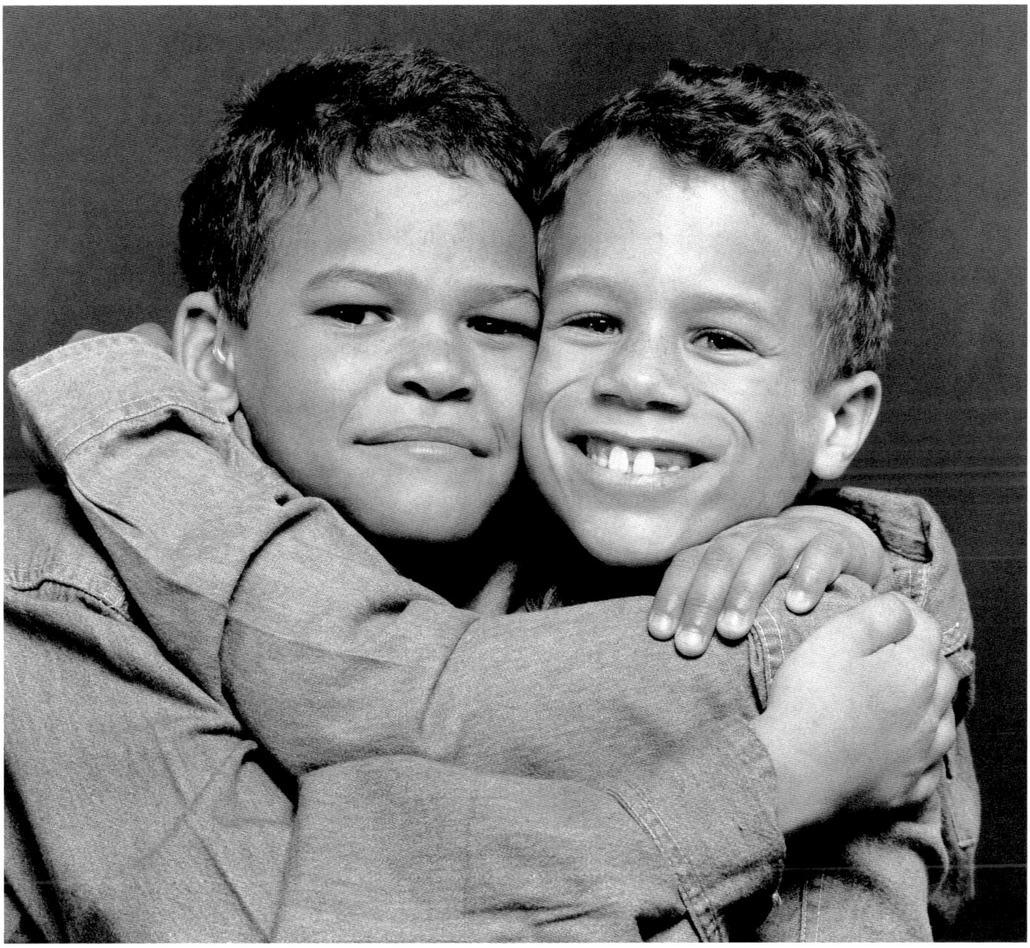

Q

our quest
for quality
of life
is riddled
with questions
just like
yours.

quagmire
(impossible extrication)
quarantine
(enforced isolation)
must I choose?

imagine
the AIDS quilt
quieting our
quivering
bodies.
yours
and mine.

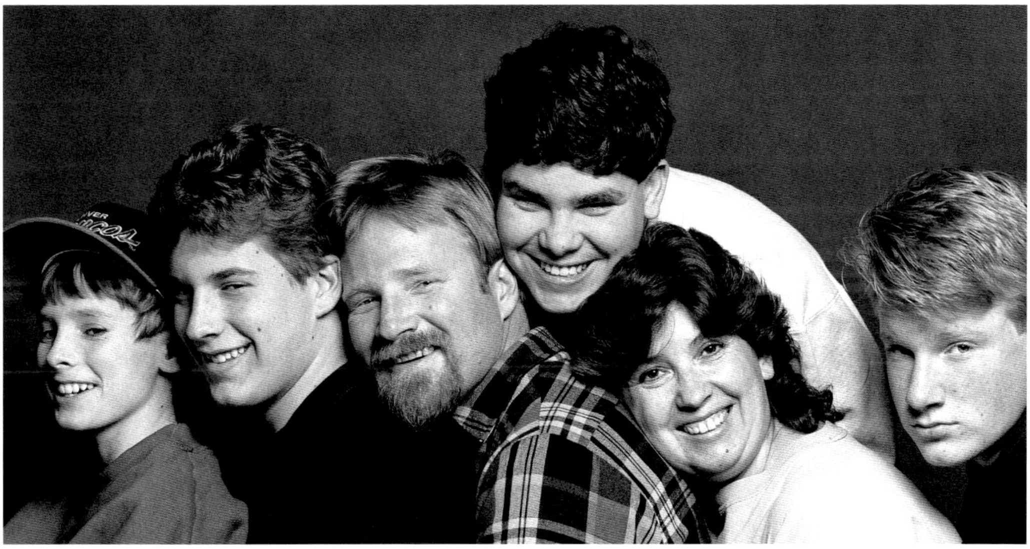

R

a padded cell
could not contain
the rage rattling
in my rebellious bones,
racing me through
my abbreviated life,
begging, restless,
ready to burst
forth in moans
as old as time.

my reality
ain't reversible.
yet.

is it risk
that got me here
or risk
that will take me
away?

someone . . .
anyone . . .
stop the rollercoaster
called life with AIDS.

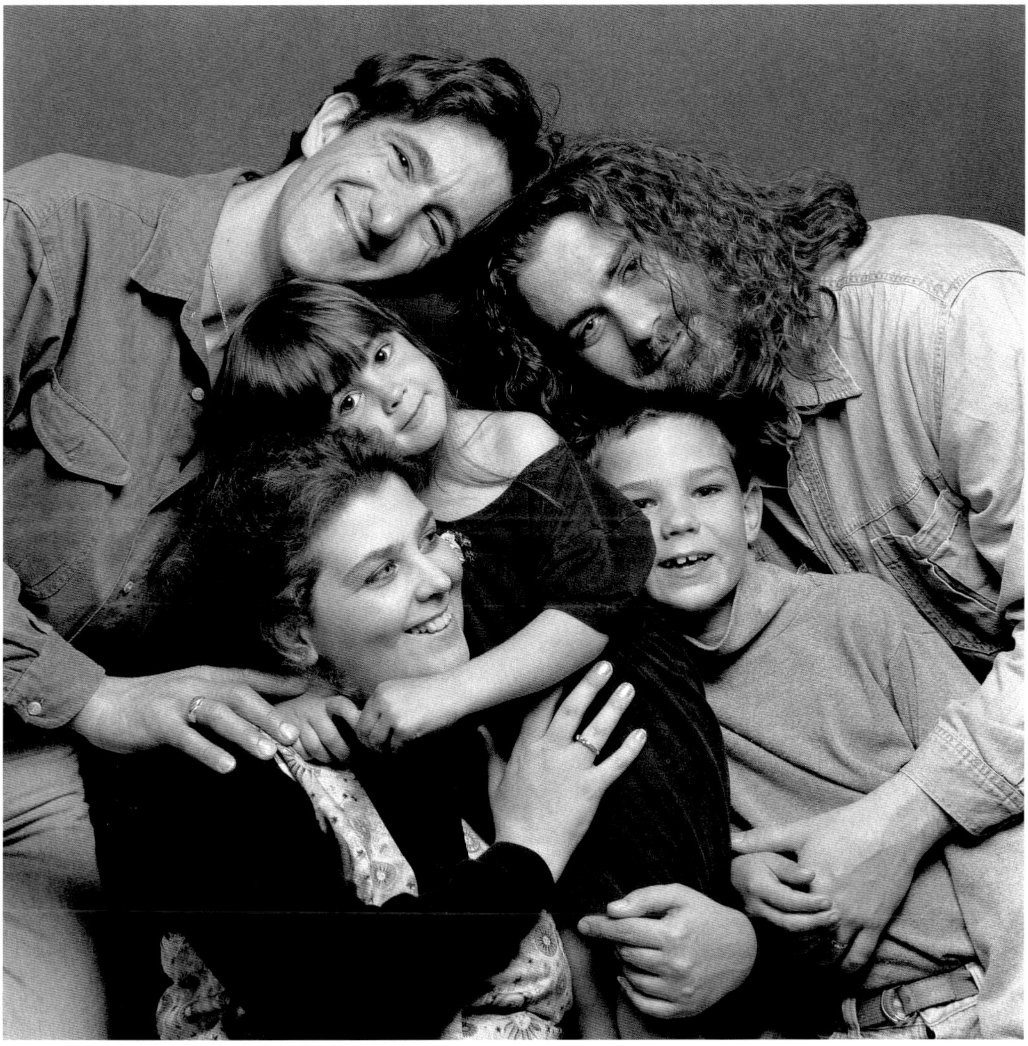

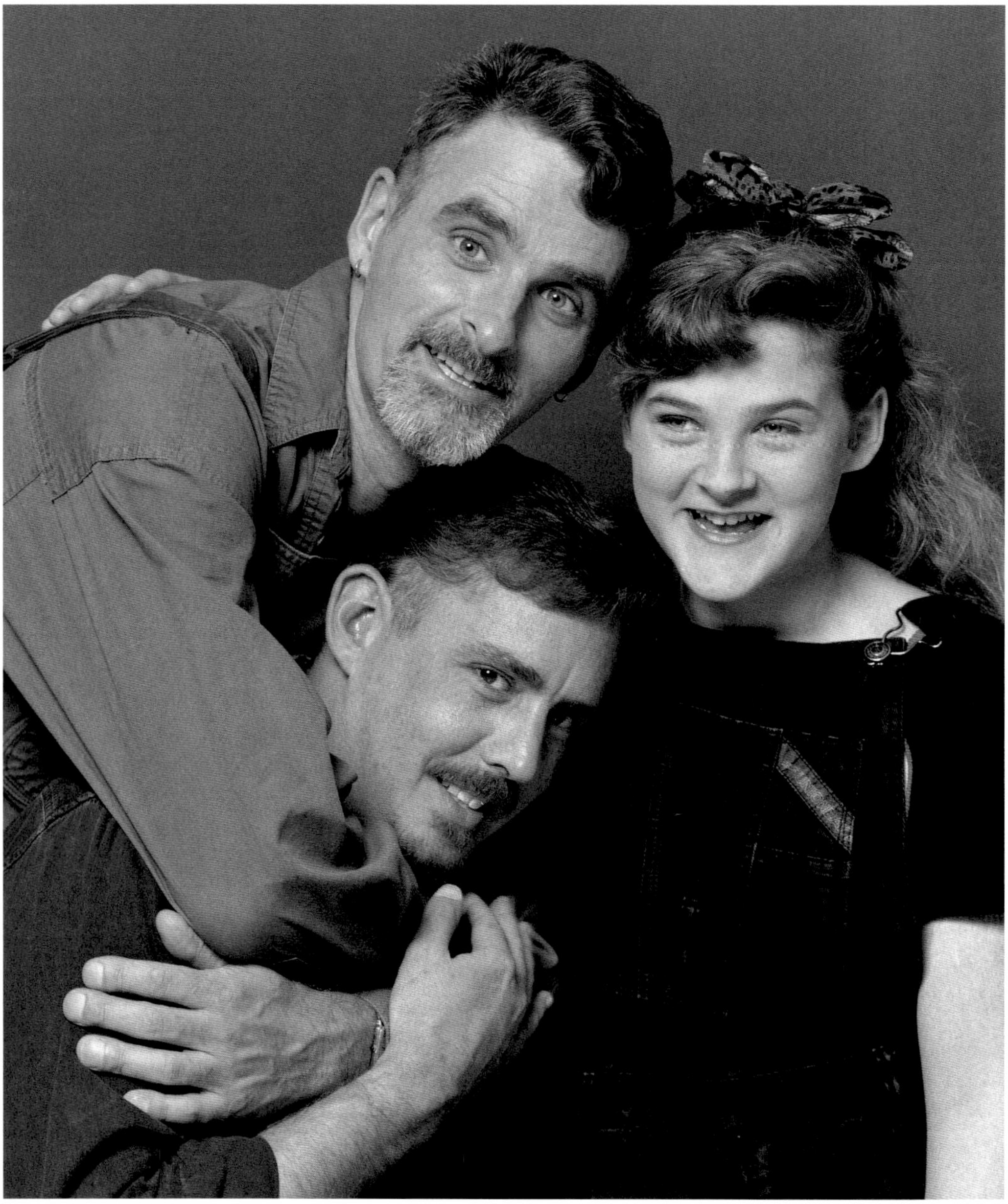

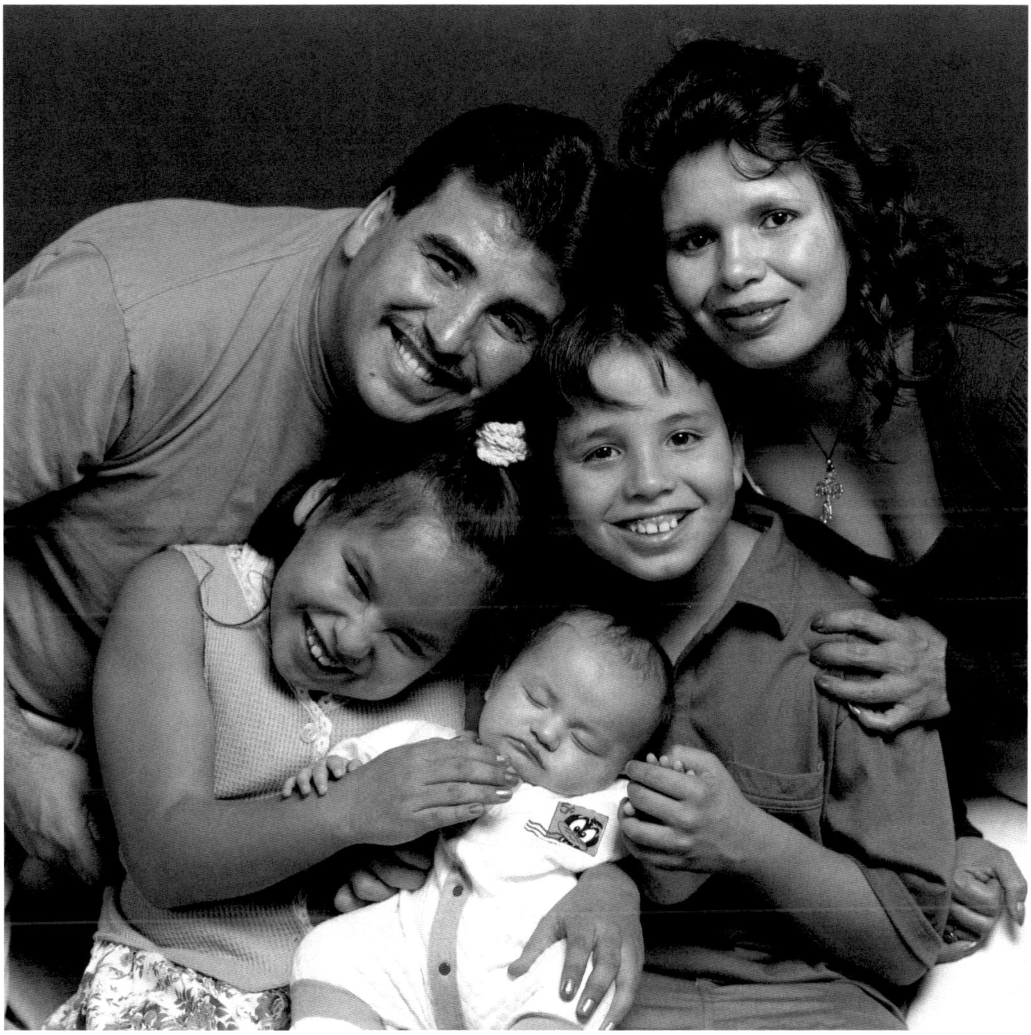

S

I am afraid that
sharing my secret
in school means saying
goodbye to friends,
hello to lonely.

AIDS cannot steal
the imprint of my child's
scent, the sheer
glory of another morning
or the smell of wet
earth as I walk
the streets in a rainstorm.
that which is sacred
has not left
but appears instead
in ways I did not know
until this moment.

some say
side effects
are the scariest.
my sadness is
the stigma
that keeps you
a stranger.

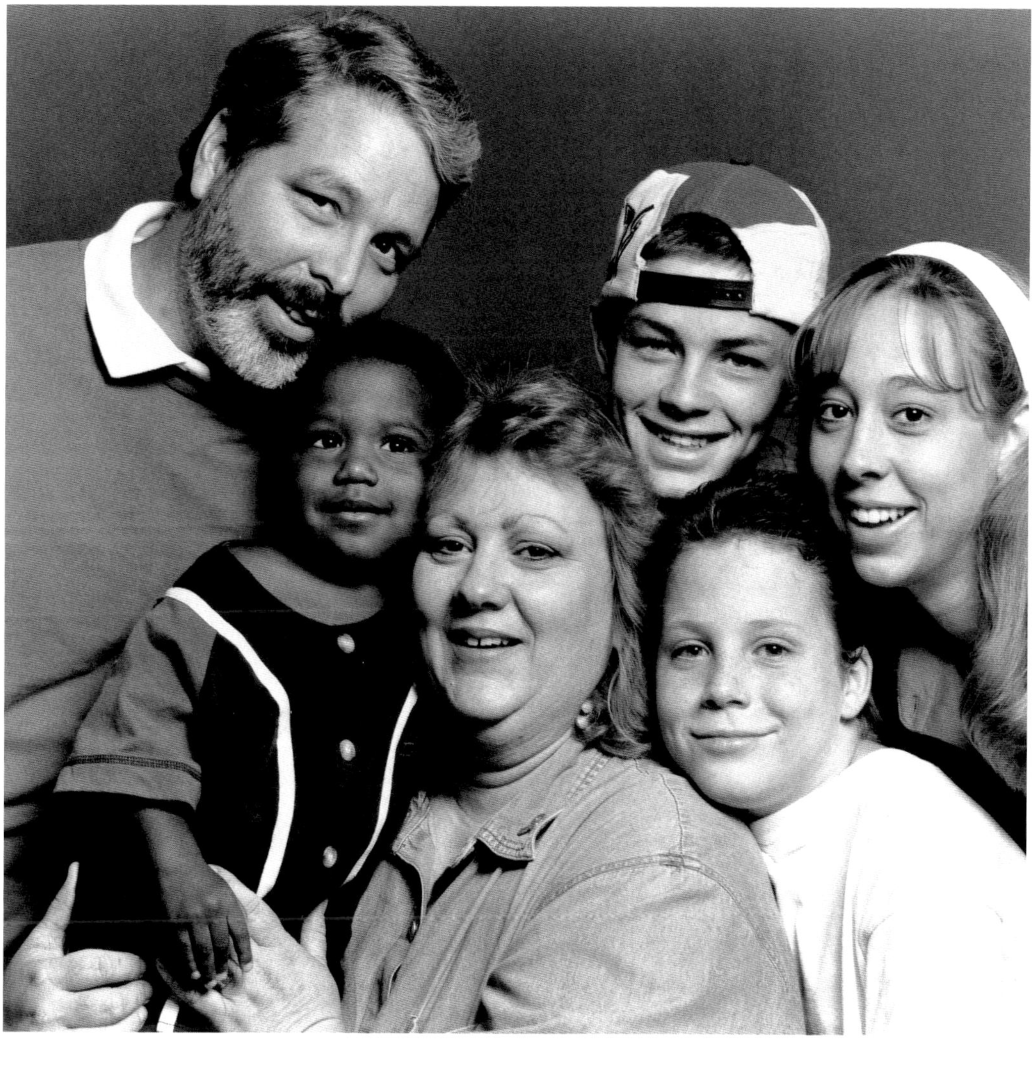

S

strength sits
in the belly of my struggle
like a fetus in my womb,
its forced silence
erupting into one
long scream
when the terrible secret
has lost its shame.

take me to shores
filled with sisters
basking in sunshine,
where struggle has ceased and
I am free
to savor the moment
my sobering secret
floats out to sea.

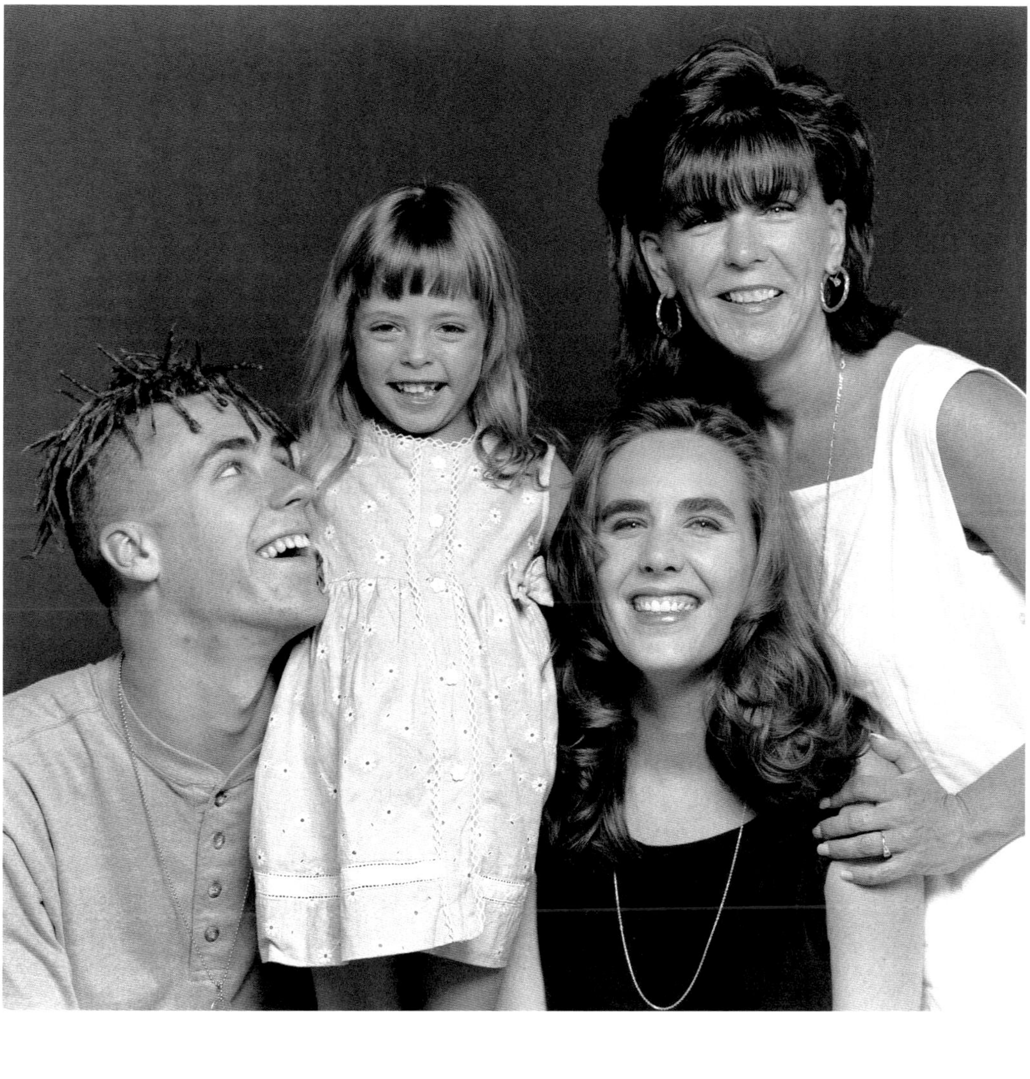

S

we can help
you save yourself
from our brand of
sickness,
syringes,
shots,
and
stigma,
but we are helpless
to protect you
from life's
surprises,
sadness,
sorrow,
and
struggle.
so you see,
perhaps we are not
so different
from one another
as you would like
to believe.

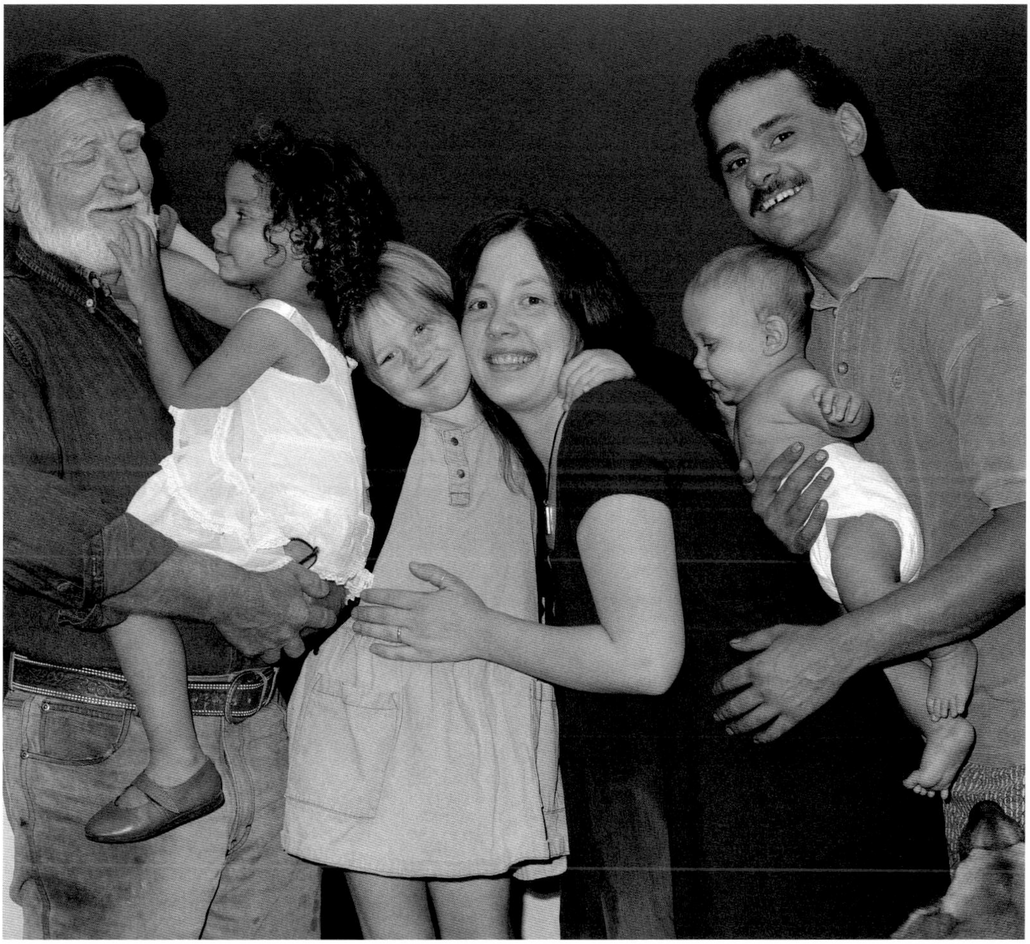

T

wipe the tears
of one of us
and you will have touched
the tears of thousands.

tenderness
matters more than
toughness.

rob your life of time
and try trusting that
terror is a teacher.

t-cells
torment
trauma
terror
tired
touch
tolerance
trust
tranquility
time

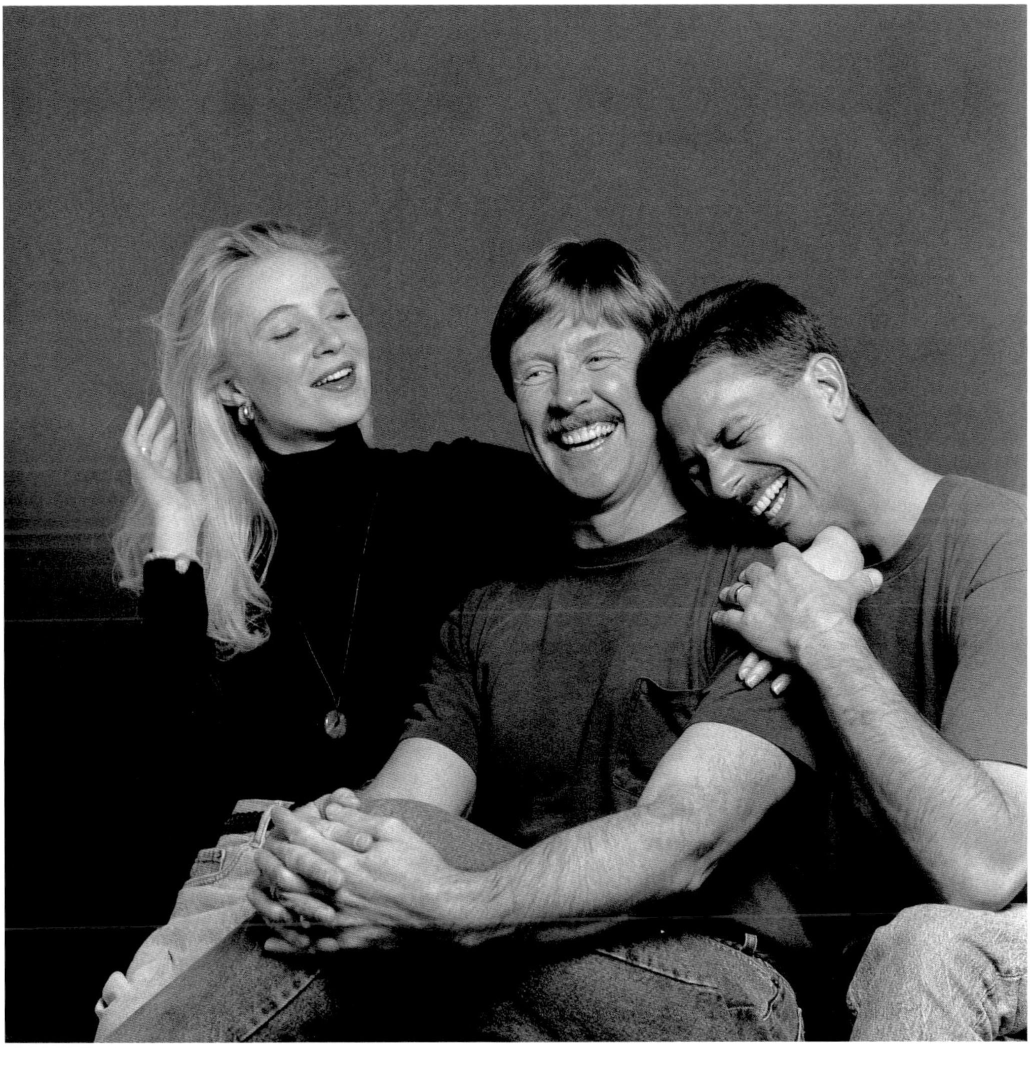

U

I am useless
at finding a way
to ignore the call of
unavoidable sadness
ringing at heart's
door, delivered
by HIV.

fear transformed
unites us in
unconditional love.

lest you consider yourself
an unlikely candidate,
this virus is universal,
democratic and ugly,
no one is immune.
take the time
to understand it.

it is unlikely a unicorn
suffers the hurt of
useless injustice.
I wish I had four legs,
two wings and
a magic horn.

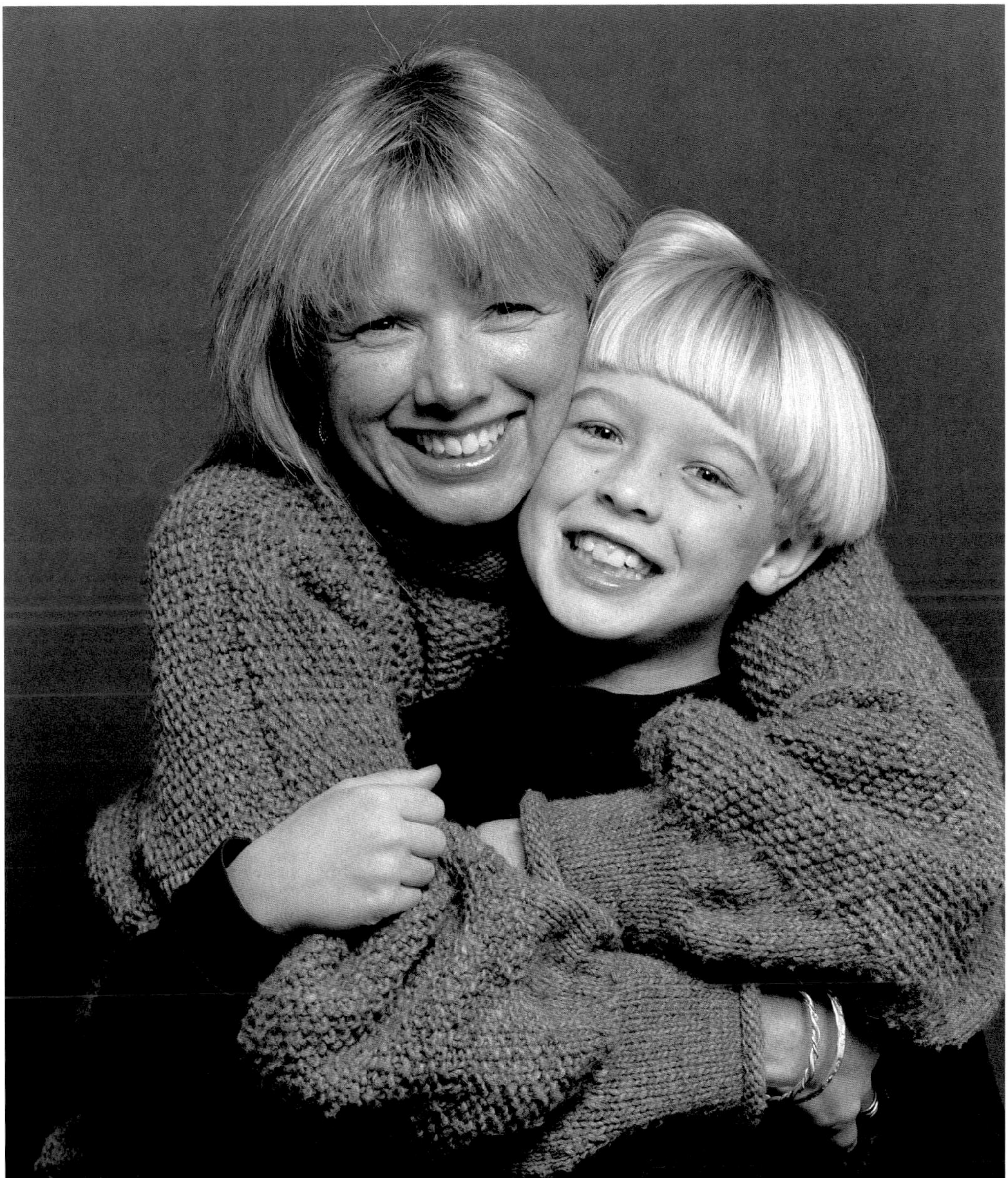

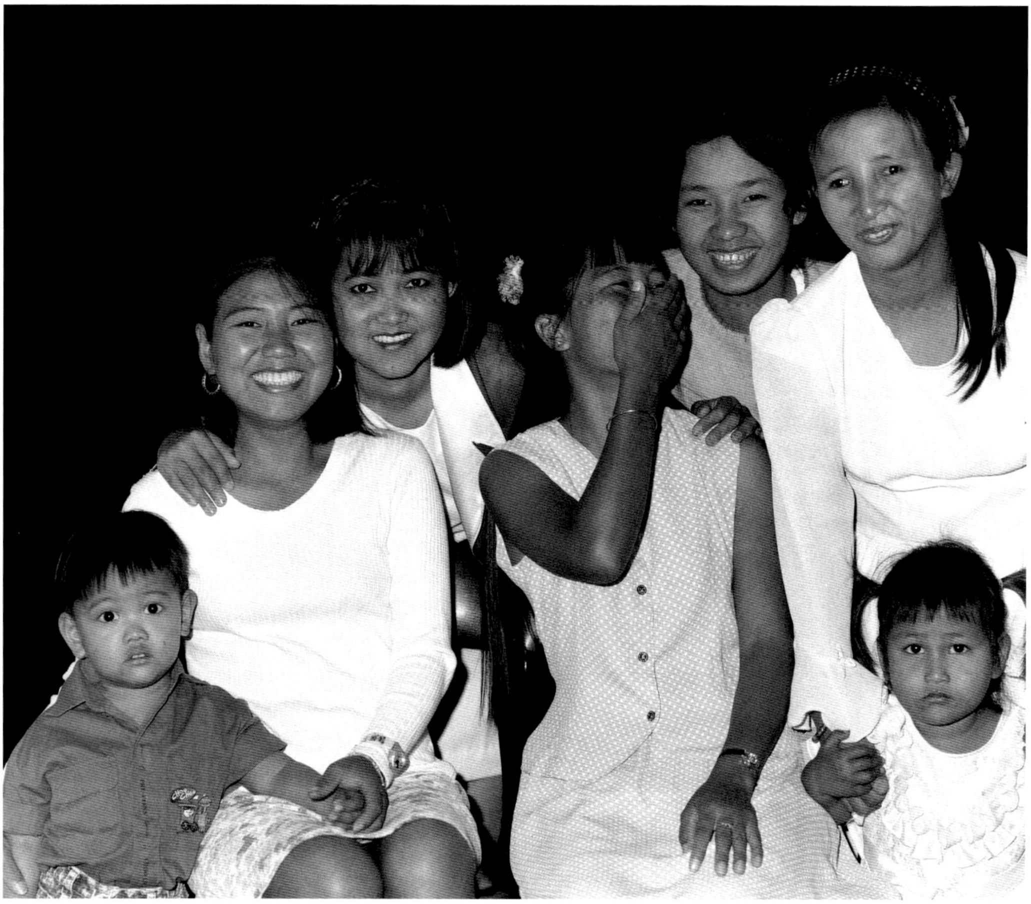

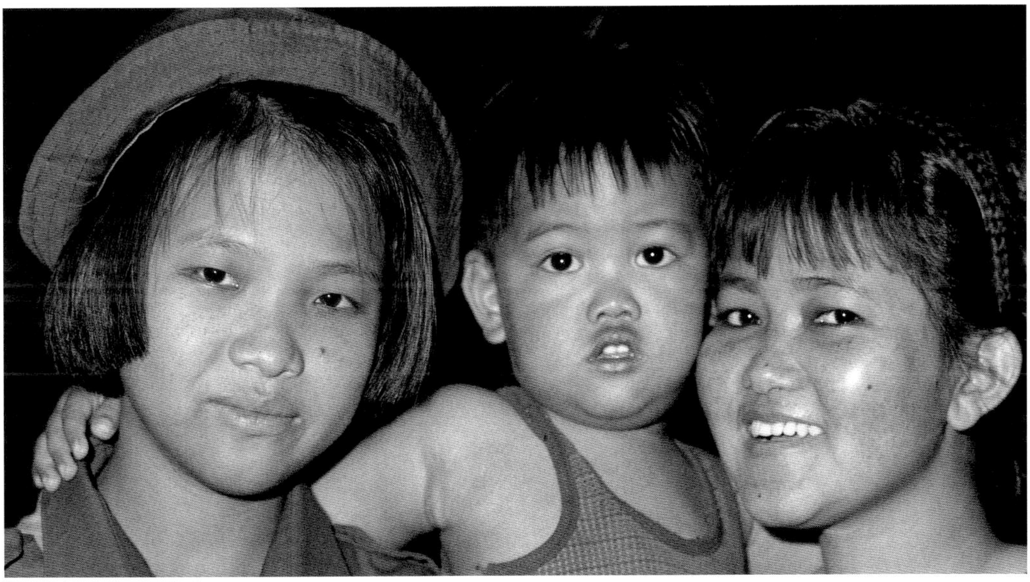

V

close your eyes
and capture the look
of a voice worn by
someone you love.

one vicious
virus and I struggle
to see myself as anything
more than a victim
of no vaccine.

a violent storm
erupted in my veins and
changed my vocabulary to
viral load,
vitamins,
and
viscosity.
what happened to
vacations?

value
me
and visit
my predicament.

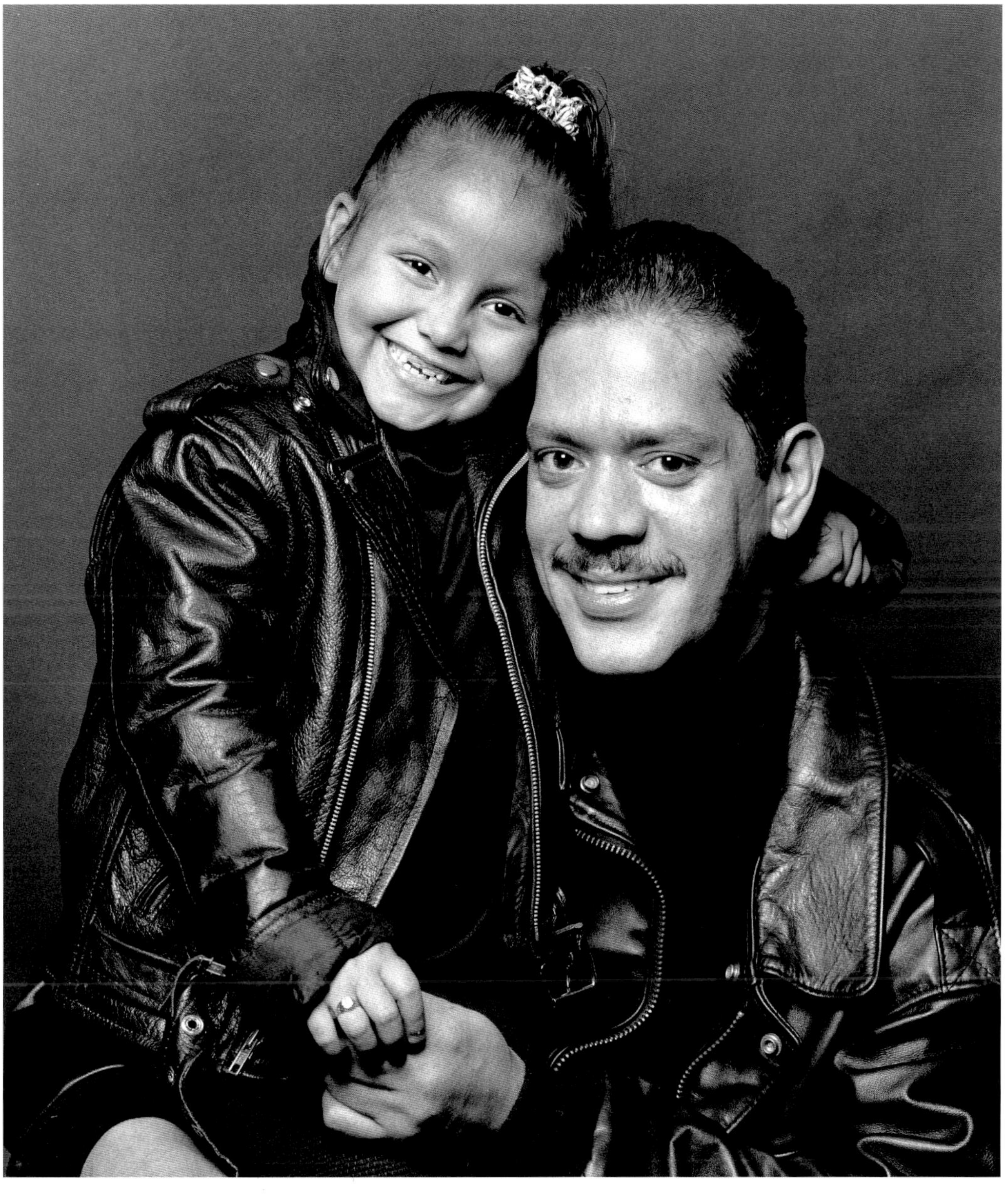

W

a pirate
named AIDS
shipwrecked my life
and buried in the rubble
a gem named
wisdom.

wake up and weep
for the wounded woman
left to wish
upon a star.

you will find me
in the waiting room
wondering
what
went wrong.

if only the witch
named worry would steal
my weakness, my weight loss,
and not my satchel
of favorite wishes.

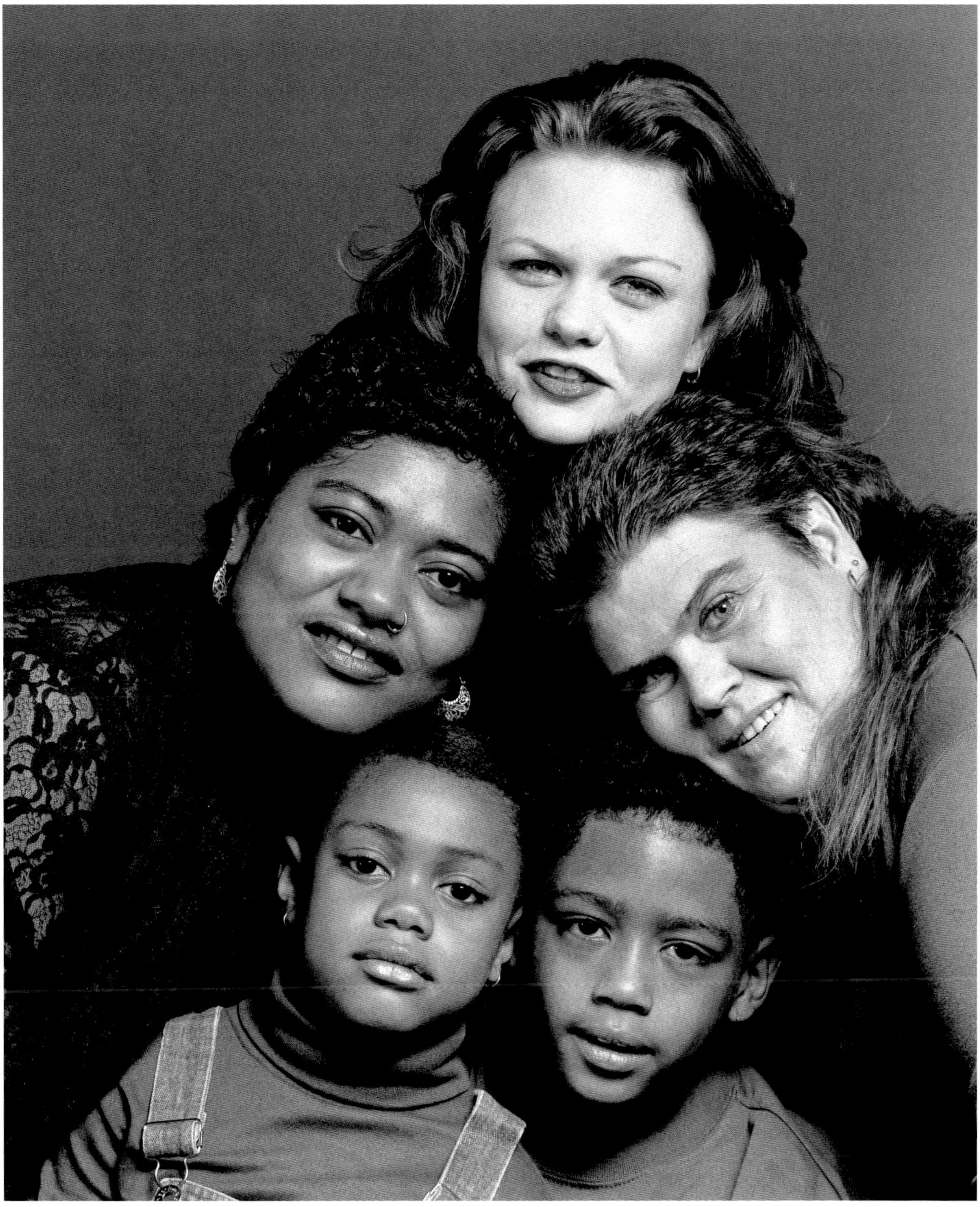

X

for one excited moment
I dreamed I had
extra time.

worried
xenophobe,
lay down your fear
and walk in my shoes.

X
HIV
out of
existence.

x x x o o o

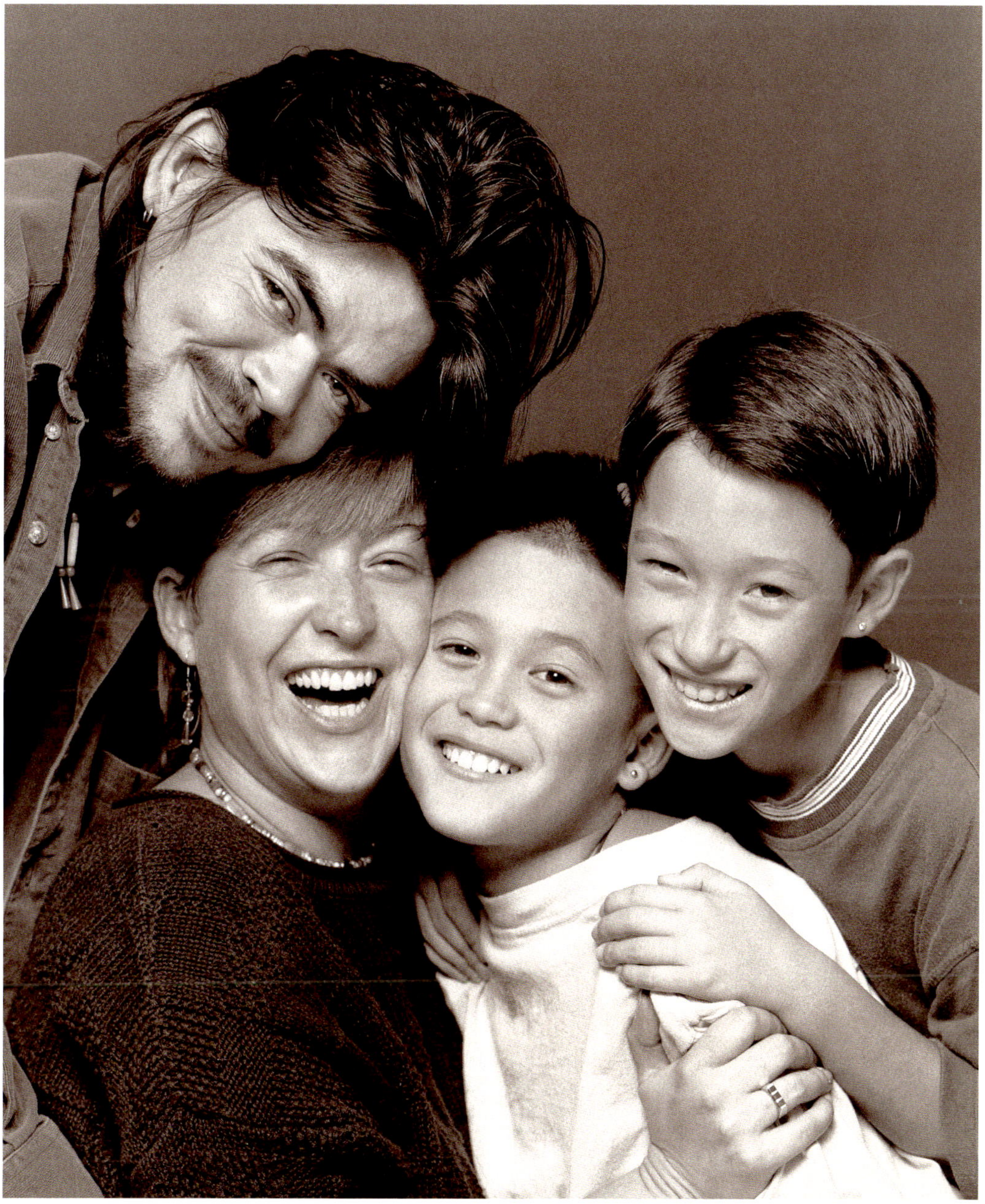

Y

yesterday
has been wrapped
in a lacy shroud of
black and white simplicity
now that nothing is
as it once was.

yucky
meds
and you
have me yelling
for understanding.

you are
a child of grace,
a spirit
filled with joy,
the greatest teacher
I will ever know.
thank you
for giving me life.

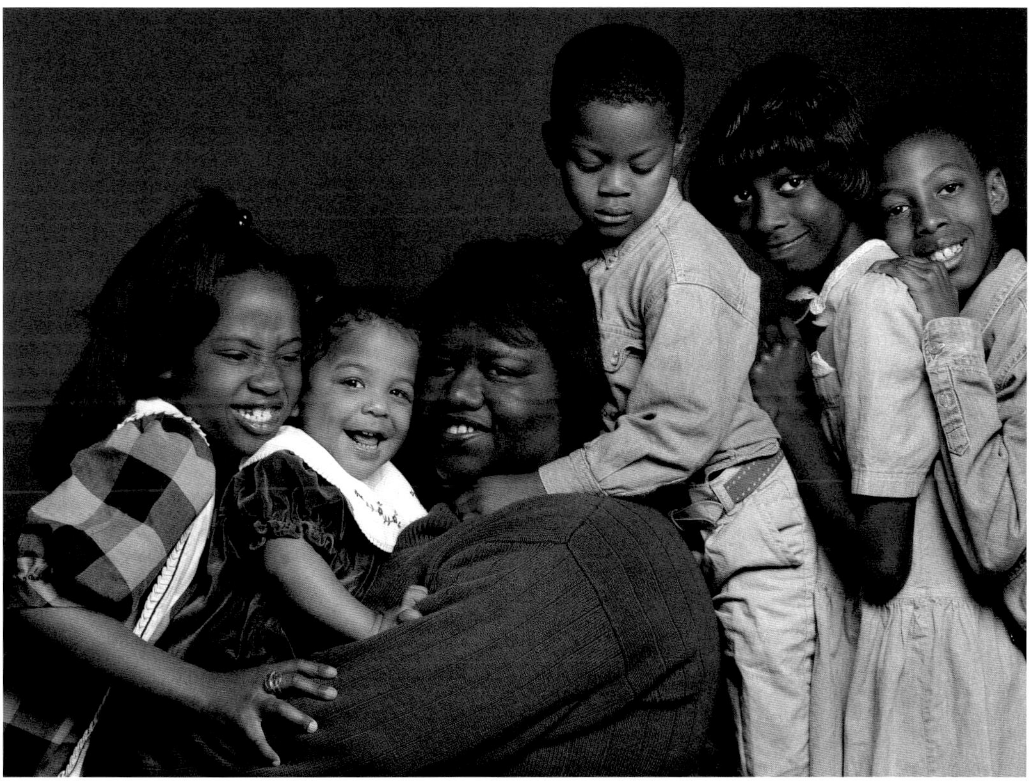

Z

we have
zero tolerance
for those who do not
care about zapping
this blasted virus.

zen
zap
zeal
zero
zone
zany
zigzag
zuberant
zippizoola.

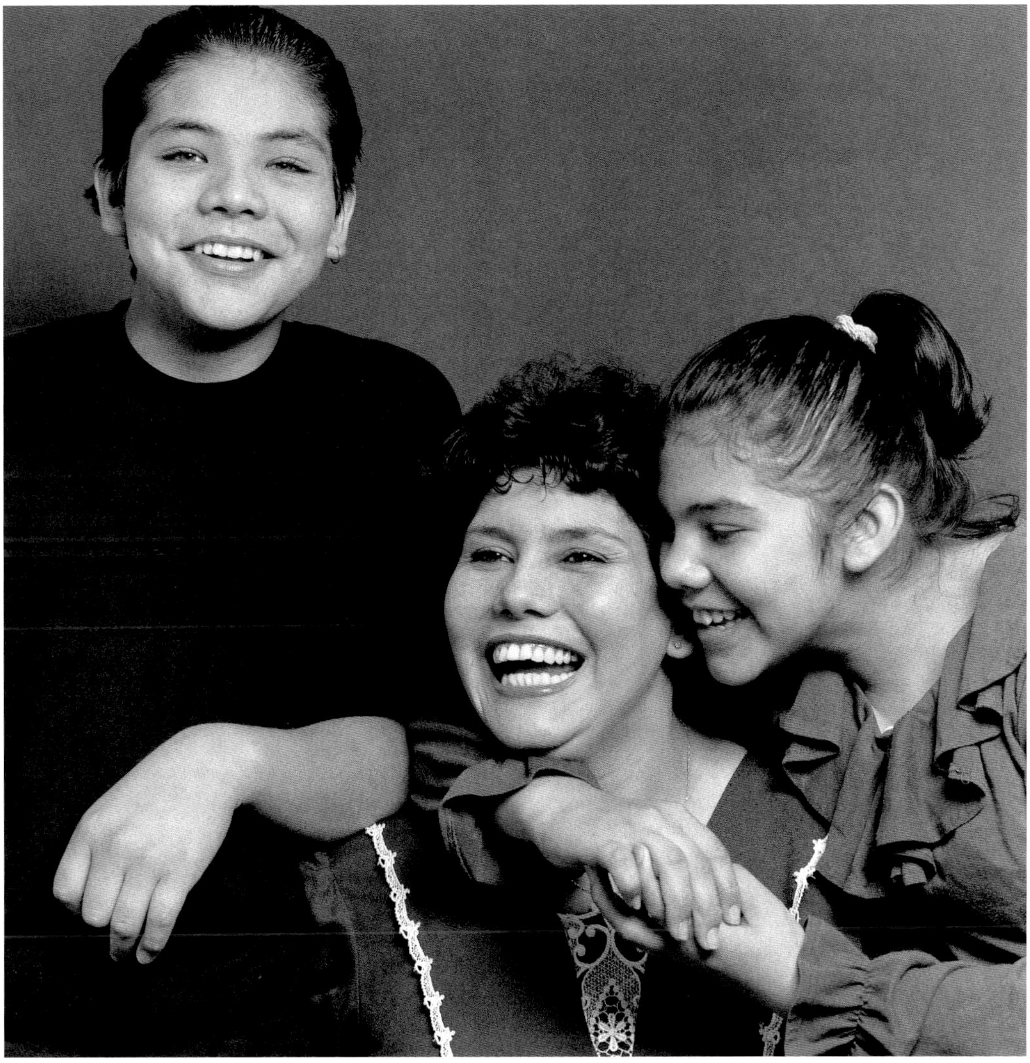

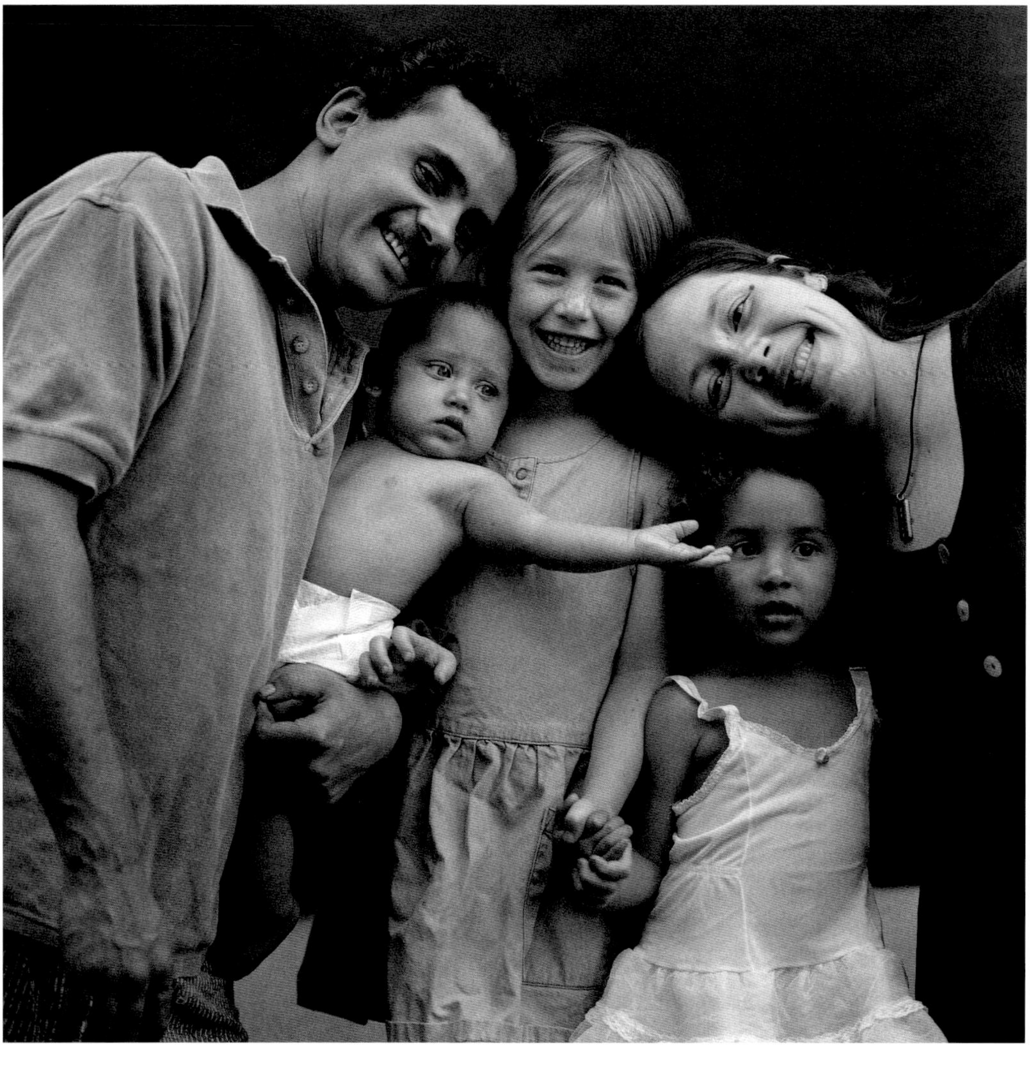

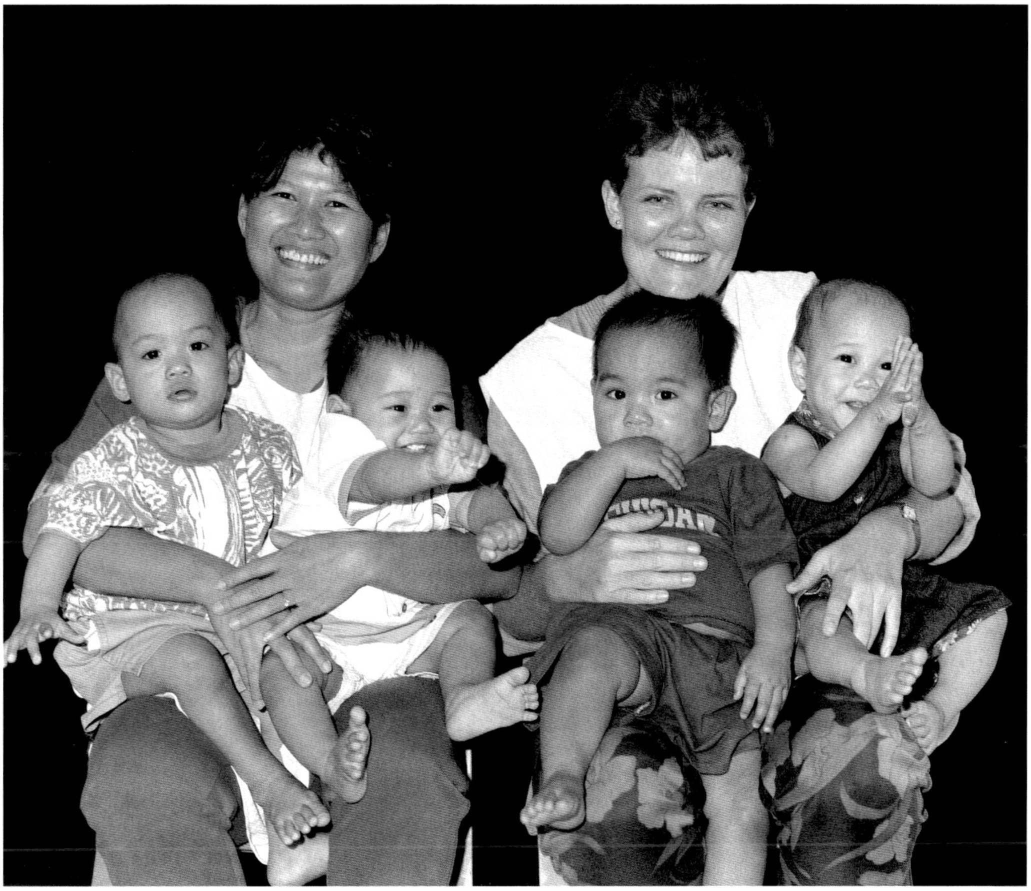

Quotes from Participants

Before I had AIDS I was very bigoted. Then I realized what a loss it was for me and how limited it made my life. – Steve

She (Mary) is a beautiful person with a lot of potential. You never think it's going to happen in your family, and you have to keep hope or faith that it will be okay. How you handle the outcome will depend on your attitude. – Cynthia on her family

Through the tough times, Randy kept his dignity. He was proud of his accomplishments, his family and his friends.
– Gary on brother Randy

I really miss my wife and my first born son, my namesake. I feel so sad. – Carlos

My daughter has AIDS. My family and close friends love her. I have HIV. We are loved. God bless all of you who just simply, beautifully love us. – Barbara

People take life for granted everyday. I do. Not! I'm constantly trying to better my heart, my mind and my soul. The greatest gift in my life is my daughter. I cherish every moment I have with Kassandra. I also want to thank my family and friends for all their love and support. I love you! – Kris

What I've learned most during my pilgrimage is that, while no two 'AIDS stories' are the same, I am a very, very ordinary woman. Each person's life is unique; AIDS does not change that so my story is, uniquely, mine. But the hurdles I've encountered in life are common to other women; the joys that make me giggle are the delights of most women blessed as richly as I am: with parents who love me, good friends who cherish me and children whose lives, I pray, will stretch far into the future. And if I've enjoyed some success in life, if I've accomplished anything that will actually make a lasting difference, it was as an ordinary person, wrestling with ordinary crises, reaching toward God for more courage than I'd have alone, and for a word of extraordinary grace. – Mary

I wanted more time. – Wanda

We responded to a need and created a home for the children who had no home, the children who live with AIDS. – Dr. Vicharn

I hope one day there will be a cure and I won't have to take the medicine anymore. – Tia

(We have) fond memories of our beloved mother and sister. Fun to be with, a great cook, a true friend who liked to wear the color red. (She was) always cold. – Loren, Andre & Irma

I always pick my words wisely because I never want the feeling that I may be judging someone and I strive for peace. – Amanda

Hope heals. – Laurie, Eliot & Robert

We are normal and have the same wishes and dreams and aspirations for our family as other people who aren't living with AIDS. Living with AIDS has really made us aware of how important our family is. – Luann & Jack

Love is meant to be shared with one another. – Mark & Gabino

In all this that we've experienced, the most important things haven't changed. 'We love each other well.' – Katie

Austin is everything that is right in this world. He is loving and kind, sweet and kissable, thoughtful, insightful, forgiving, precious beyond belief. If I could be like anyone, I would be like him. When I asked Austin what he would like others to know about him, he simply said 'that I am a nice person and that I care about others.' – Lorraine

Ryan chose to educate. He was calm and didn't complain, even in the worst of times. He worried about whether or not everyone else would be okay. When people made hurtful comments, he would say 'now mother, they're just uneducated.' – Denise

My name is Darin BenFord, Jr. I have a brother and a sister. My brother's name is Justin BenFord and my sister's name is Brizjette Williams. In October my father, Darin D. BenFord, Sr., passed away from AIDS. It was a hard day for me because I was really close to my father. – Darin

My name is Justin BenFord. I have a brother and sister. My brother's name is Darin BenFord, Jr., and my sister's name is Brizjette Williams. Me and my brother's father had AIDS and he passed away on October 3, 1995. That was a real sad day for me and my brother. – Justin

Life is what you make it. There's always good in everything. – Hydeia & Patricia

I'm an extremely proud Dad. – Frank

Hope, love and healing. – Agape House

I brought the light of unconditional love, bravery and wisdom to a blessed family. Don't cry for me; I have wings and I'll see you all soon. – Clarice (in the words of Kathy)

We're not going to let AIDS destroy one minute of our lives. We're going to do everything we can while we can. – LaRue

AIDS is certainly a mixed blessing. We experienced a loving closeness and an urgent desire to pour ourselves into 'family.' – June & Mike

I am a good kid. My parents love me, Ladessa my mom, Michael my dad and David my uncle. We have a big family. – Matthew

I feel very bad for my two dads, but I feel since I've been living with them, I've gotten closer to both of them and learned more about the HIV/AIDS virus. I'm learning more as days go by. – Angela

Racism hurts. – Anonymous

I want people to know I'm not going to hurt them and I just want to be friends. – Tyler

I have a family—they love me and make me happy. I make their world better. – Alison (in the words of Joanne)

The unconditional love in our family helps us live with AIDS instead of die from AIDS. – Kevin & Ren

I am someone who likes to make people smile or laugh. – Bob

We live too fast and we die too slow. – Mary

When I sing together with Poppy, it makes you happy. – Ileana

Always remember through the sorrows, struggles, tears, smiles, laughs and hugs, each day is a blessing. – Jody

I am nice. I am ten years old. I like stuff like earrings because I have one. I like jewelry and stuff like that. I am very nice and very smart. I am good at math. – Anonymous

Karmen has filled our life with beauty and love. Thank you for sharing your smile with us. Love, Mommy. – Arta

Sometimes I cry myself to sleep because I am scared that my mom will get sick again, and she might die this time, and when I wake up every morning, and see her smiling at me and telling me she loves me, my fears go away because we are living with AIDS, not dying. – Maritza

I thought no one in my family could get AIDS or HIV until my mom told my sister and I that she had tested positive. I still remember how mad I got, but I am somewhat over it now, and I still love my mom and enjoy all my time with her. – Martin

List of Participants who chose to have their names included:

Frank Ackerman & Byron Pendley with Nathaniel Ackerman
Cynthia Alvidrez & Mary Hope Suarez with Reynaldo Gallegos, J.J., Crystal, Monica & Ruben Alvidrez and grandchild
Arta Banks with Nehemiah, Nicole, Kathryn, Kaleb & Karmen Banks
Marc Barocio & Gabino Jacobo with Chelsea & Maria Barocio
Luann Bauer & Jack Patterson with Mai Bauer and Anthony, Brandon & Kristina Patterson
Mary Wilson Blanton with Casey Blanton
Kellie Bock & Chris Haselton with Katie Haselton
Pat Broadbent with Kimberly Davis, Briana & Hydeia Broadbent and Patricia Washington
Bob Brown & Steve Caldwell with Jillian Caldwell
Barbara Bryon with Doriann Bryon
Laurie & Robert Cohen with Eliot Cohen
Lesbia Cruz with Andre & Loren Cruz/not pictured sister Irma Abalos & husband John Ignatius, niece Lina Ignatius and nephews Johnnie & Marquez Ignatius
Mary Fisher with Max & Zachary Campbell
Kris Foerstner with Kassandra Adamson/not pictured partner Robert Howard deceased
Israel Gerena with Ileana Gerena/not pictured daughter Sirerra Gerena deceased
Lorraine & Tim Gregory with Lucas Gregory and Austin & Avery LaMar
Anita Jones with Randy Jones
LaRue Kelley with Breana, Tyree, Tenaya & Bryon Kelley
Tim Kelley with Angela Kelley and Bruce Charley
Wanda Laboy & Carlos Lebron with Carlos & Onyx Lebron/not pictured daughter Yaricali Lebron
Kathia Luengo with Maritza & Martin Sanchez
Dee & Ron Morgan with Tia & Kevin Morgan
Kathy Foos Nuanes with Clarice Foos-Brockington
Stephen Prince with Roxie & Cody Prince
Michael Riter with Ladessa, David, Matthew & Heaven Cremeens
Donie Rivera & Carol Torres with Donie & Crystal Torres and Cecil Rivera
Amanda Rosas with Jamie Lynn & Melissa Rosas
Carlos Ruiz with Gustavo Ruiz
Denise Sheridan with Ryan & Garrett Sheridan
Cindy & Larry Small with Tonya, Trenton, Tyler & Bubs Small/not pictured son Tim Small
June & Michael Tuff with Andy, Troy, Jason & John Tuff
Marie Veasley with Darin & Justin BenFord
Joanne Venn with Alison, Oriana & Zach Venn
Joannie Williams & Darling Chinn with Karie Williams and Ugene & Kanisha Chinn
Kevin & Ren Worden with Sasha, Nyssa & Nason Worden and Larry Worden
Women & Children of the House of Love, Chiang Mai, Thailand
Staff & Children of Agape House, Chiang Mai, Thailand
Staff & Children of Dr. Vicharn's orphanage, Chiang Mai, Thailand

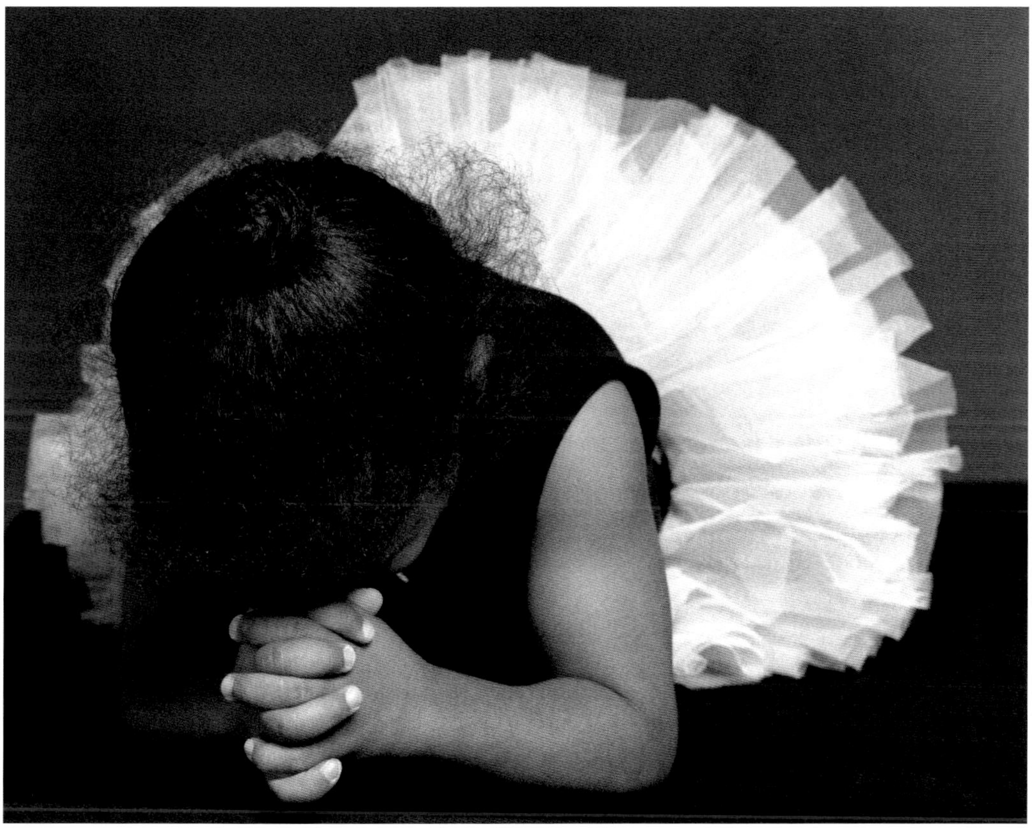

Your Turn

The following pages contain every word submitted for this book. They come from mothers, fathers, sons, daughters, sisters, brothers, spouses, partners, stepmothers, stepfathers, stepchildren, stepbrothers, stepsisters, grandmothers, grandfathers, grandchildren, aunts, uncles, nephews, nieces, cousins, adopted children, birth children, guardians, and caretakers who have become family.

Contributors represent a range of sexual orientation. There are those who contracted HIV through contaminated blood factor in treatment for hemophilia and other diseases, those who are infected due to mother-child transmission, and others who contracted HIV through sexual behavior and/or IV drug use. The photographs include people who have died, people who speak freely about living with HIV, and people who have been living in secret and found the courage to come out with publication of this book.

We invite you to read their words and explore the ways each of us is connected to one another through our humanness. When the time is right, add your words to the pages, fill the frames with a favorite photograph, memento, quote, keepsake or poem. Personalize your book. Make it your story, your legacy. There is no finer gift we give one another than to allow ourselves and our truth to be seen, understood and remembered.

A

abandoned, abolish, abolishment, absolute counts, abstinence, acceptance, admire, adults, afraid, age, aggressive, agony, AIDS, AIDS–it's everywhere, alive, Almighty, alone, always, always, always Allie, always remembering to take meds, amor, anger, answers, anxiety, anyone can get it, appetite, appreciate, aspiration, avoid, awful, AZT

B-my friend, babies losing their parents, baby, bacteria, bacterias, Bactrim, bad, bad tasting medicines, baffled, battle, bedstricken, beginnings, being sick, being thankful for every minute, being there, belief, believe, belonging, beloved, best friends, bet, beware, bias, biopsy, bizarre, blame, bless, blessed, blessings, blood, blood work, body, boldness, bonito, bored, boring, bothersome, brain involvement, bravery, breakthrough, brother, Broviac, Brownie the pony, bummer

Camp Heartland, cancer, care, careful, caregivers are wonderful, caring, caring for others, caring doctors who help, carino, carpe diem, cat scans, catheter, cells, child, children, chilling, clinics, CMV, community, compassion, concern, confidence, confidential, confusion, contagious, coping, coughing, courage, cranky, create, cry, crying, cuddling, culture, cure, cured, curious, cut, cuteness

D

daddy, dangerous relations, day-by-day, DDI, dear dad, death, death of friends, death (wife), deceptive, delight, denial, depression, desilucion, desperate, destroyed, destruction, devastate, devastated, diarrhea, different, difficult, dignity, disaster, disclosure, discrimination, disease, distracted, doctor, doctors, don't die, don't know, dose, drugs, dying

E

ear infections, early morning meds, easy does it, earthshaking, education, effort, elegant, elephant, eliminating, embarrassment, emergency, end (whenever that might be), enemy, energy, enjoying what is, envious, epidemic, epitaph, ER – home away from home, era, eradicate, error, esperanza, eternity, eulogy, everlasting, everybody, everything, evil, exciting new medicine, exhausted, exhaustion, expectation, experience, experience, experimental, experimental, experimental protocols, experiments for new treatments, eye exams

F

faces, fail, faith, fallacy, familia, families, family, fatal, father, fathers, fatigue, favorite, fear, fever, fevers, fight, fighting as a family, find a cure, fire, flames, flight, forever, forgetting you even have this disease, forgiveness, fortunate, freedom, friend, friends, friends that you make in the hospital, friends – they hold us up and keep us going, fright, frightened, frightening, being made fun of, fungus, future

G

gaining, gamma globulin, ganas, gathering, gay, GCSF, GCSF shots, genocide, getting scared, girls, giving, God, God is loving me through this, gone, good, goodness, got me! grace, grateful, great, great doctors and hospital staff, great doctors, nurses, and social workers, great friends and family, grief, grieving, group support, growing, growing stronger through the years, growing up, growth, Grumpy & the 7 dwarfs, guilt, gusto – trying to pour weeks of life into every day, gut check

H_2O, ha, happiness, happy, hate, having to lie, headaches, heal heal heal me, healing, healthy, heartbreaking, hearts, heavy, hell, help, helpful, helping, helpless, hemophilia, Henry, hidden, hiding, hiding the truth from the rest of the world, HIV, hijos, holding on, honesty, hope, hospital, hospitals, hot, how come, hugs, hurt, Hydeia

I

ignorance, ignorance breeds denial, illness, imagination, immune system, immunity, important, Indiniver, infection, infections, informing, infusion, infusions, injections, injustice, inquisitive, insidious, inspiration, instability of life, insult, insure, intelligent, intense, interno, invisible, IQ tests, irreversible, isolated, isolation, IV, IVIG, IV's

Jacob, jaded, jail, jamming food into your mouth, Jasmine, jeopardy, jerked around, Jesus, jinx, jokeless, jokes (AIDS), AIDS jokes, jokingly, jolly, journey, journey to stay alive, joven, joy, joy of life, joyful, Jr High School (scared to go), judgments that people make, juggling medicines with normal life, juggling your time, jugular, jump rope, just one day, justice kangaroo, kaput, karma, keep the HIV virus from spreading, keeping alive, keeping secrets, key, kids, kids helping kids, killed, kill, killer disease, killing, killing the virus, kind, kindless, kindness, kiss, kisses, mommy kissing my owie, knowing, knowledge lagrimas gears, lapiz, laughing, laughter, Laylie, learning, leaving, left, leopards, Lesbia, life, lightning, lions, liquids, live live live and love love love me too! live life while you can, living, living on the edge, living with HIV, loneliness, lonely, love, love from my family, love—only unconditional love can defeat AIDS, loving everyday, lying, lying to others

M

mad, madness, magic cream, Mai, Make-A-Wish, making friends, malice, Mary, meal, medication, medicine, medicine being constantly taken, medicines, medis, meds, mellow, memorials, memories, method, midnight snacks, miedo, mindset, miracles, misery, mom, moms, money, more love, mother mothers, mountains to conquer, mourning, MRI, much prevention needed

N

naptime, narrow-minded, nausea, neatness, nebulous, need, needles, needs, nervous, never knowing what's going to come next, never say never, never say not me, new findings, new medicines, new pills, new treatments, nice, nieto, night sweats, nightmare, Nintendo, no, noble, nobody, no-no, noodle, Norbert, normal, notorious, nourish, now, nurse, nurses

O

oasis, ocular, odd, ominous, one day at a time, open, opening, opening up, openness, operate, operation, operations, opinion, opportunistic, opportunistic infections, opportunities, oppressed, optimistic, optimistic attitudes, option, options, organize, orphan, Orrie my sister, oportunidad, ostracize, ouch! our problem is here—let's heal together, outpatient clinics

P

paciencia, pain, painful, past, patience, PCP, peace, peace–a constant desire for the peace that HIV/AIDS interrupted, peers, people, perspective, pharmacy, pills, Pinocchio, play in life safely ...please, please peace, pneumonia, porta cath, positive, positive, positive(HIV+), being a positive person, positively, potential, prayers, praying, praying for someone to break through and find a cure, presents, prison, private worries, problems, progress, prospective, protease inhibitors, protect, protocol, protocols, puke, purpose quality, quality of life, quarantine, feeling queer, queer person, quest, questionable, questioning, questions, questions about why I'm not at school, questions? let's find answers, quiet, quiet time, quiet times, quietly, quilt, donated quilts, quit, quite, quivers

R

race, race for the cure, races, radical, rainbows, rational, reality, rebellion, recognizing faces, rejected, rejection, relief, relief when something's over–my favorite feeling, remember, reordering, rescue from meds, resolving, respect, respeto, responsibility, rest, resting, restricting, retina, Retrovir, reverse the statistics, Rifabutin, right, rights, rise, Rise-N-Shine, risks, rollercoaster, rotten, rude

S

sad, sadness, salud, save yourselves! let our experiences help you, savor each moment, school, scream, secrets, secrecy, self, sensitive, sex, sexy, sharing, shots, sick, sickness, side effects, silent cries for help, silliness, singing, sinusitis, sisters, sleepy, social workers, socializing, sorrow, sorry, stigma, strength, struggle, stupid, stupid illness, suck, sucks, suffering, sun/son–both full of warmth and shine brightly in our life, sunshine, support, supportive, surprises, sweet, swollen, syringe

T

t-cell count always being unpredictable, t-cells, talking, teaching, tears, tears of pain, technology, teen group, temperature, temperatures, tenderness, terrible, terror, tests, there is hope, thrush, time, tired, TLC, today, together, told, tolerance, tomorrow, torment, tormented, toughness, Toys R Us, trading secrets, tranquility within myself, traumatic, travails, treatment, treatment, treatments, trisdesa, trust, trusting, truth, twilight zone, twisted, Tylenol, Tyler

U

ugly, ultimate, unavoidable sadness, uncertainty, uncomfortable, unconditional love, understanding, unexplainable, unfair, unhealthy, unicorn, unify, union, united, unity, universal, universal precautions, unjust, unknown, unpredictability of the virus, unprotected sex, unwillingness of others to learn about this disease, upper respiratory infections, use precautions, useless

V

vacation from pills, vaccine, validation, valor, value, valve, vase, veins, vertigo, very cute, vicious, victim, victory, victory–over shame and ignorance, victory–every new day is a victory, vile, violence, violent, viral load, virtue, virus, viruses taking over people's lives, viscous, vision, visit me when I'm ill, sad and happy, too! vitamins, vulnerable

W

waiting, waiting for a better treatment, waiting room, wake up, want, wanting, war, Washington, D.C., waste, ways, weakness, weeping, weight loss, well, we're in this together, what, wheelchair, when, where, who, why, will, willingness, willpower, wisdom, wisely, wish, wishes, wishful, wishing, wishing for a cure, wishing I could tell others, wishing star, witch, withdrawn, women, wonder, wondering, working, working hard to keep up, worry, worst, wound, wrong

X “x”, x-am, x-citement, x-disease, xHIV out of existence, xenophobe, xeno-phobia, x-ray, x-ray photographs every 6 months, x-rays, x-tent, x-tra time

Y – me?? yah yah, yearn, yearning, years, yell, yelling for support, yelling for understanding, yelp, yes! we need you! yesterday, you, young, young, young people, youngsters, youth, yucky medications, yucky medicines, yucky meds

Z

zzzzzzzz (getting plenty of sleep), Zach my brother, zany, zap that blasted virus, zarconian felozie (sounds good), zeal, zealous, zebra, zen, zerberts, zero, zero cells, zero t-cells, zest, zest for life, zesty, Zidovudine, zigzag - my counts, my health and my life, zigzagging temperatures and appetite, zipper, zippizoola, Zovriax, zone, zoo, zoom, zuberant

About The Children's Legacy

The Children's Legacy, a 501(c)(3) nonprofit, was founded in 1987 by Denver photographer Katy Tartakoff. Our mission is to provide opportunities for children and families faced with life-threatening illnesses to celebrate their lives with photography, art and writing. We are committed to inspiring change in the public sector by sharing the families' photos and stories through the development of educational materials and photography exhibits.

In the past eleven years, hundreds of families whose children are living with life-threatening illnesses like cancer and AIDS have been served at no charge by the Legacy. Thousands more have been touched by Legacy publications including *My Stupid Illness, Let Me Show You My World* and *Burned and Beautiful* (Tartakoff; 1991), as well as *An Alphabet about Kids with Cancer* (Berglund & Tartakoff; 1994). We are thrilled to add *An Alphabet about Families Living with HIV/AIDS* (Lee, Tartakoff, Blanton & Wiener; 1998) to our stable.

In the past year, the photography and art of The Children's Legacy has been on display in several venues including the Denver Art Museum, Denver Museum of Natural History, the Joslyn Museum of Fine Art, Omaha, NE, and the Community Visual Arts Association Center, Jackson Hole, WY. The Children's Legacy was named the 1997 recipient of El Pomar Foundation's prestigious Spencer and Julie Penrose Award as the Outstanding Nonprofit in the State of Colorado.

Everyone has a story to tell. Through the sharing of our stories, we connect with one another. The stories of families who live with a life-threatening illness teach us about daily life with a terminal virus, surgical scars, an artificial limb, a bald head. The work of The Children's Legacy is life-affirming. Families are honored and celebrated for their truth. Photography and art are the canvas for them to tell their stories and to share those stories with anyone willing to enter a world of courage and hope. To celebrate our lives, regardless of duration and circumstance, is to honor the gift that each of us has been given, the gift of life.

To learn more about The Children's Legacy, or to order a Legacy publication, contact:

The Children's Legacy
P.O. Box 300305
Denver, CO 80203
phone: 303.830.7595
fax: 303. 860.9648
e-mail: tclphoto@aol.com
web site: http://members.aol.com/tclphoto